FUNDING
THE
CURE

HELPING A LOVED ONE WITH MS
THROUGH CHARITABLE GIVING TO THE
NATIONAL MULTIPLE SCLEROSIS SOCIETY

Martin M. Shenkman, CPA, MBA, JD

Demos

Library of Congress Cataloging-in-Publication Data
Shenkman, Martin M.
  Funding the cure : helping a loved one with MS through charitable giving to the National Multiple Sclerosis Society / Martin M. Shenkman.
    p. cm.
  Includes index.
  ISBN-13: 978-1-932603-48-4 (pbk. : alk. paper)
  ISBN-10: 1-932603-48-4 (pbk. : alk. paper)
  1. Multiple sclerosis. 2. National Multiple Sclerosis Society (U.S.) 3. Charitable bequests. 4. Endowments. I. Title.
  RA645.M82S54 2008
  616.8'34—dc22

                                                                      2007028485

DISCLAIMER: Neither the publisher nor author provide through this book any legal, tax or other professional advice. Readers are cautioned not to take any action in reliance on the materials presented in this book without first consulting their own professional advisers. Tax situations vary significantly from individual to individual. Tax and other laws change frequently, and there are significant differences in state laws, so professional guidance is essential to implement any of planning ideas in this book. The National Multiple Sclerosis Society (NMSS) has not endorsed or approved the contents of this book, or the recommendations contained herein, and has no responsibility for the contents of this book.

SPECIAL ORDERS: Special discounts on bulk quantities of Demos Medical Publishing books are available to corporations, professional associations, pharmaceutical companies, health care organizations, and other qualifying groups. For details, please contact:

Special Sales Department
Demos Medical Publishing
386 Park Avenue South, Suite 301
New York, NY 10016
Phone: 800-532-8663 or 212-683-0072
Fax: 212-683-0118
E-mail: orderdept@demosmedpub.com

Book design by Steven Pisano
Made in the United States of America
07 08 09 10 11   5 4 3 2 1

Dedicated to Eileen, Larry, Joey,
and so many others suffering from MS,
but mostly, to my beloved wife Patti,
whose beauty, strength of character,
and sense of humor
continue unabated.

WACHOVIA
WEALTH MANAGEMENT

Dear Reader:

Wachovia is delighted to underwrite a portion of the cost of this wonderful book titled *Funding the Cure*. Wachovia has been a long-time supporter of the National MS Society. Our employees have given generously of their personal time and financial resources, and have been active participants in MS Walks throughout the country. We welcome this additional opportunity to support the efforts of such a worthy cause.

Wachovia is committed to supporting the National MS Society in its quest to find a cure for multiple sclerosis, while helping those living with MS and their families to deal with the impacts of the disease. Our professional staff of financial planners, investment advisors, and charitable giving specialists is readily available to help prospective donors, their families, existing advisors, and the National MS Society to implement a wide array of charitable giving techniques. Through planned and deferred gifts, such as charitable lead trusts, charitable remainder trusts, and other planning techniques, we are confident that, working together, we can help to raise significant funding to support the efforts and the wonderful work of the National MS Society.

At Wachovia, we have known the author, Martin Shenkman, for many years as both an excellent attorney and prolific writer of legal books that make difficult topics easy to understand. We value his friendship, professionalism, and respect for Wachovia's ability to assist his clients with their estate and charitable giving plans. Marty's passion for finding a cure for multiple sclerosis is contagious, and we look forward to partnering with all of you in this vital quest.

Sincerely,

Donald E. Lewis
SENIOR VICE PRESIDENT
Wachovia Wealth Management

Foreword

THE NATIONAL MULTIPLE SCLEROSIS SOCIETY (the Society) is committed to building a movement by and for people with multiple sclerosis (MS) that will move us closer to a world free of this disease. Through our 50 state network of chapters, we fund MS research, provide services to people with MS, offer education programs for health care professionals, and further advocacy efforts on behalf of people with MS.

Planned gifts, such as those discussed by Martin Shenkman in this book, are vital to ensuring that the Society meets the needs of those affected by MS both today and in the future. Deferred gifts made today ensure that the Society will maintain momentum in the fight against MS and continue providing much-needed services, programs, and research until the day we find the cure.

Every person and every family affected by MS has an important story to share. I want to thank Marty for sharing his story and for all he has done to advance the mission of the Society. His passion for and dedication to the movement against MS is evidenced in his stream of innovative ideas and his drive to see them realized. It would be impossible to move the Society's mission forward without the willingness of people like Marty to share their support, personal stories, time, and incredible talents.

MS stops people from moving. The Society exists to make sure it doesn't. Join the movement at nationalmssociety.org.

Joyce Nelson
PRESIDENT AND CHIEF EXECUTIVE OFFICER
The National Multiple Sclerosis Society

Foreword

I HAVE LIVED WITH MULTIPLE SCLEROSIS since 1984. At the time, I was finishing up seven big years as the character Squiggy on the television show *Laverne and Shirley*, and anticipating a life doing what I love best—making people laugh. Life was sweet with my wife Kathy and daughter Natalie, but then MS changed everything.

As my life changed, everyone in the family realized that we would need to be a team and look out for and care for one another in new and different ways. We also knew that we would do everything we could to put an end to this disease. I desperately want to stop its insidious progression in my body, and I want to spare others from the pain it has caused me and those I care about.

But there is good news now and helpful strategies available to meet the special care needs of those, like myself, who have MS—and still promote the research and services of the National MS Society that will bring us closer to a world free of MS.

To find out how you can do this, I recommend that you review the stories and strategies Marty shares in this book, and then talk with the Society or the person who helps you with financial planning. It's easy. People like me are doing it, and people like you should be too.

Why? Because we all care too much about our families and about MS not to get involved. And because there are so many people counting on us. Thanks for giving us the insights to help anyone facing healthcare issues, whether it is ourselves or our families, and with the gifts we make helping our global MS family as well.

David Lander
ACTOR

About the Author

MARTIN M. SHENKMAN, CPA, MBA, JD, is an attorney in private practice in Teaneck, New Jersey and New York City.

Mr. Shenkman has been quoted in: *The Wall Street Journal, Fortune, Money, The New York Times*, and other publications. He has appeared on: *The Today Show, NBC Evening News*, CNBC, CNN-FN, and other broadcasts.

Mr. Shenkman is author of thirty-two books and more than seven hundred articles. His books include: *Living Wills and Health Care Proxies; Estate Planning After the 2001 Tax Act; Homeowner's Legal Bible; Divorce Rules; The Complete Living Trust Program; The Complete Probate Guide; Beneficiary Workbook; Estate Planning After the 1997 Tax Act; Starting Your Limited Liability Company; The Complete Book of Trusts; Investing After the New Tax Act; Real Estate After Tax Reform; Real Estate Tax Planner; Shopping Center Leases: The Tax Impact; How to Do Tax Planning with Depreciation, Amortization and Tax Credits; The Accountant's Role in Divorce; Marketing for CPAs;* and *Estate Planning Step-by-Step*.

Mr. Shenkman has served as contributing editor to: *New Jersey Lawyer, The Journal of Real Estate Finance, Real Estate Insight, Commercial Leasing Law & Strategy, The Journal of Accountancy, Real Estate Accounting and Taxation, Shopping Centers Today*, and others.

He is a member of the American and New Jersey Bar Associations, various accounting and financial planning organizations, and numerous charitable organizations.

Mr. Shenkman received his BS from Wharton School, MBA from the University of Michigan, and law degree from Fordham University School of Law. He is admitted to the bar in New York, New Jersey, and Washington, DC. He is a Certified Public Accountant in New Jersey, Michigan, and New York.

Contents

CONTENTS

CHAPTER 4: DIFFERENT ASSETS CAN BE USED TO HELP FUND THE CURE

CONTENTS

CHAPTER 5: MEET PERSONAL GOALS WHILE FUNDING THE CURE

CHAPTER 6: TAX RULES FOR CHARITABLE GIVING

CHAPTER 7: WHAT YOU CAN DO NEXT

CHAPTER ONE

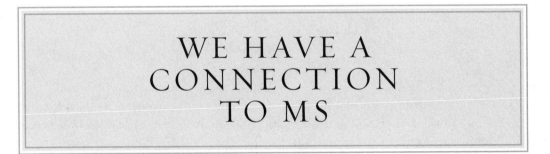

WE HAVE A CONNECTION TO MS

I HAVE A CONNECTION to multiple sclerosis (MS), and if you're reading this book, it's likely you do as well. Your connection will be unique to you, as mine is to me. But whatever your connection to MS, hopefully this book will help you find ways to address your personal connection to MS, help you accomplish financial and other goals, protect and benefit yourself or a loved one, all while benefiting the National Multiple Sclerosis Society (the Society) and furthering its goal—our goal—of ending MS and finding a cure. But to find a cure, we need to fund the cure. That is the task at hand.

> *The time is short, the task is great…*
> *the master is demanding*
> —Ethics of Our Fathers 2:17

For those living with MS, the urgency to find new treatments, methods of repairing myelin and axonal damage, and providing local programs and services has never been greater. The task is indeed great. The damage caused by MS changes lives. The master is demanding. MS affects millions worldwide. The complexity of the disease is daunting. The mechanism by which T cells penetrate the blood–brain barrier, communication between oligodendrocyte and myelin, and communication between myelin and the underlying axon increases the need for more sophisticated magnetic resonance imaging (MRI) technologies to assess axonal damage, and so much more. The challenges to ending MS are many. Our help in providing funds as donors, and our help in guiding and encouraging others to make gifts and bequests to help finance research and other activities, is essential to those affected by MS, and to the millions more who love and care about them.

My Connection to MS

My wife was diagnosed with MS, an "incidental finding" it was called. But when someone you love is diagnosed with MS, it's anything but incidental. First there was the shock of the diagnosis. Everyone deals with the shock differently. My wife cried on my shoulder for days. We immersed ourselves in reading more than a score of books, scouring the Internet for articles, attending seminars, consulting with experts, and more. I discovered (yes, for us it was a discovery) the National Multiple Sclerosis Society. We sought information. In short order, we attended the Society's annual convention. We discovered much more than just a wealth of information to help us plan my wife's course of treatment, and our new lives. We discovered an entire community of caring and involved people, all motivated by the same goal: supporting and helping those with MS while endeavoring to find a cure. It is an understatement to say it was reassuring to know that the safety net of Society knowledge, research, and many caring people is there. The burden is easier to bear when you have those to share it with.

We sought to get involved because anything we could learn gave some certainty and comfort in the world of unknowns that MS creates. We probably also got involved because a diagnosis of MS made us both feel so helpless, and making a contribution of time, money, and effort combats this feeling. Perhaps your contributing to the Society, or your helping encourage others to contribute, will help empower you, if you or a loved one is affected by MS. This book will guide you with scores of ideas on doing so.

Funding the Cure

There are many ways to give to the Society and help fund the cure for MS. You can encourage or guide others to give in scores of ways. This book does not focus on describing complex tax and legal methods of charitable giving. It's a book about people. It's about you and people you care about. Rather than exhorting you to give or to get others to give, we'll share with you some of the things that we've done. Different approaches may work for you or other prospective donors, but hopefully these illustrations will give you a better understanding of the many possibilities available. You don't have to limit yourself to a particular approach; there is usually no single or "right" approach. The goal should be to develop a plan that meets your personal needs and objectives, the needs of your loved ones, all while benefiting the Society and the MS community and maximizing tax benefits for you.

Simple Pledges

We made pledges payable over several years. Perhaps you have or will do so as well. Making a pledge payable over several years can help the Society budget for specific projects you wish to support. It provides an example that can encourage others to make larger gifts. If your finances don't permit a large gift at one time, making a commitment that you pay out over several years is a great compromise.

Bequests and the Pillars of Society

We updated our wills naming the Society as a beneficiary. For us, it was a way of showing a permanent and long-term commitment to help fund the cure. By making a bequest to the Society, we both became "Pillars of Society" members, the membership group for those making a bequest to the Society in their wills. It's easy to do. The next time you amend or update your will, add a specific bequest to the Society: "I give and bequeath the sum of $_____ Dollars to the National Multiple Sclerosis Society, which is presently doing business at 733 Third Avenue, New York, New York 10017." Your estate planner can discuss variations on this simple bequest and alternative ways to fit it within your plan.

When dealing with the frightening prospects of what MS can bring, the physical and cognitive impairments are most feared. But MS creates financial difficulties as well. For us, as for so many living with MS, work efforts had to be significantly limited. Yet making a bequest in a will is a method of making a commitment, demonstrating your support, but without any cash outlay while you are alive. A bequest (donation paid under your will following death)is a great way to give back, even if you're grappling with the financial challenges of MS.

Our participation as Pillars will hopefully encourage others to make bequests as well. Perhaps you can join us in that endeavor. It is not just the amount of the bequest that is vital, but the fact that you make the commitment. The greater the number of Society Pillars, the greater the likelihood of obtaining new bequests and even new current gifts. The more bequests and gifts, the greater the funding for MS research that can lead us to the cause and cure.

Insurance Planning

Multiple sclerosis forces everyone affected to rethink all their personal planning. This includes estate planning documents, investments, and so on. Specific changes are warranted to address the unique issues that MS creates. For us, the question was: How could I revise our planning to best protect my wife financially and legally? Financial protection could mean ensuring an adequate cash flow if MS symptoms progress. It can also mean addressing the loss of employment as the consequences of MS take hold. Among other steps, legal protection can include preparing a power of attorney (which designates an agent to manage assets and take legal actions if you cannot), a revocable living trust (which provides for more comprehensive management of assets than a power of attorney), a living will (a statement of health care wishes), a health care proxy (which designates an agent to make health care decisions), all specifically tailored to address the issues MS creates. How could I best help the Society in its search for a cure while still protecting my wife? For now, as for many with a new diagnosis, a substantial current gift is difficult because resources must be preserved for the uncertainties of the future.

How could I conserve financial resources in the face of the financial impact of MS and loss of wages and, at the same time, make a meaningful commitment and contribution? I purchased a permanent (not term) life insurance policy, to be owned by the Society, and for which the Society is a beneficiary. For a rather modest annual premium, which is fully deductible as an income tax charitable contribution, I've endowed a future gift of more significance than I felt I could otherwise presently do. I made a commitment which in itself was rewarding to us, because it was another means of taking affirmative action in light of the helplessness that MS created for our family. It was another means of helping to fund the cure.

The gift of a life insurance policy, however, was just another one of the long list of reminders of MS's ever-present impact. It was a bittersweet endeavor, because my wife cannot for now obtain life insurance because of her diagnosis.

Hopefully, my insurance plan will provide an example to encourage others, perhaps even you, to make a planned or major gift to help fund the cure. If you have a spouse, child, partner, friend, or other loved one living with MS, your endowing a major gift through an insurance policy can also be a wonderful way to show your solidarity and support to them.

This Book

Each of us has our own unique ways to help the Society in its mission. This book is another way we've endeavored to help fund the cure. While the primary goal of this book is to guide others in making significant gifts to the Society, all royalties on this book have been pledged as a donation to the Society, and all royalties will be donated directly by the publisher to the Society. Whatever special skills or abilities you have can certainly be used to help. Whatever your personal situation and financial circumstances, there are ways for you to contribute and make a difference.

How This Book Is Organized

THREE KEYS: PEOPLE, ASSETS, GOALS

Each of the steps we've taken to help fund the cure, and many, many more, will be explained below. For you, the first steps are to:

- Identify who it is you're trying to help. Chapter 3 focuses on the different people you can help in the process of funding the cure.
- Determine what resources and assets you have available for planning. Chapter 4 reviews how many different types of assets can be used to help fund the cure. Don't worry if you don't personally have the resources. By helping those you know or meet identify planning ideas, you can indirectly help fund the cure.
- Address other goals you have. Chapter 5 shows you how you can achieve various personal, family, or other goals while supporting the Society and the MS community.

Your goals may include planning for your retirement, or helping a child with MS plan for her retirement, helping pass a business onto your heirs, or providing for the education and medical costs for your grandchildren. All these, and many more of your goals, can be integrated with steps to help fund the cure.

TAXES

Taxes! Because our tax system is so complex and costly, few charitable gifts are made without planning to maximize the tax benefits. Part IV reviews many of the tax benefits you can achieve for income, gift, estate, and generation-skipping transfer (GST) tax. The income tax is the tax on your current earnings. The gift tax is a tax on any large gift (over $12,000/year) that you make to family or friends. The estate tax is a tax on the value of assets you own at death. The GST tax is a tax on assets you give or bequeath to grandchildren or later descendants. Charitable donations to the Society can help you save on any or all of these taxes.

GLOSSARY/INDEX

Jargon abounds, so we've provided a glossary and index to help ease the way through the planning ideas. Also, all technical terms are defined in the text when first used. Finally, more detailed definitions are available at www.laweasy.com.

The goal of this book is to offer you a wealth of planning ideas, each of which can result in a charitable gift of some sort to the Society to help fund the cure. The goal is to explain and illustrate charitable planning in an understandable fashion, for those living with MS, or like me, who have a loved one with MS. The planning is different from standard planning because dealing with MS, as you well know, changes everything. This book is not intended to be a treatise on charitable giving. Your personal accountant, attorney, financial planner, and other advisers—as well as the expert volunteers and staff of the Society—can all help guide you through the maze. But if this book can give you and others a practical idea to begin helping fund the cure, we'll be a step closer to achieving our goals.

Chapter Summary

We all have a connection to MS. Whether you live with MS, have a friend or loved one affected by MS or, from the standpoint of compassion and concern, wish to help the millions worldwide who face the many challenges of MS, we all have a connection to this disease. We all share a common goal. Our mutual connection should motivate us all to help fund the cure for MS. A myriad of ways are available in which you can:

- Achieve many of your personal planning objectives
- Benefit yourself or a loved one who has MS

- Do so using whatever resources you have
- Obtain potentially significant tax benefits

This chapter has endeavored to encourage you to consider charitable planning to help fund the research efforts and other benefits and programs of the Society—to help fund the cure. The following chapters will show you how.

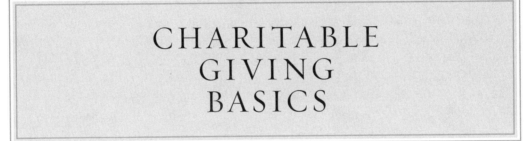

CHAPTER TWO

CHARITABLE GIVING BASICS

THIS CHAPTER INTRODUCES THE BASICS of charitable giving. many approaches can be taken. Writing a check is but one method. More complex approaches will enable you to tailor a charitable giving plan to meet more detailed and personal objectives.

The National Multiple Sclerosis Society (the Society) is dedicated to finding a cure for MS through carefully funded research efforts, while also supporting local programs and services to those with MS, their caretakers, and loved ones. While the Society continues to be successful in raising both awareness and funds through events such as MS Walks and MS Bike Rides, a myriad of additional giving opportunities can move us toward a world free of MS. Carefully planned gifts to the Society can also help the donor (whether it is you, a family member, or another) achieve important personal, income tax, estate tax, and other benefits. This book explains many of the strategies you can use to make gifts to the Society, or help others to do so. To understand these strategies, this chapter provides an overview of the many ways charitable giving can be planned and understood. The purpose of this chapter is to help you think about charitable giving in broad and flexible terms, to understand some of the basic concepts and terminology, and to begin to set the framework for how you (or those you know) may specifically help fund the cure using the techniques discussed in Chapters 3, 4, and 5. The more technical tax concepts are left for Chapter 6, which will be easier to understand once you've identified some of the planning ideas you wish to pursue (or as an alternative, you can merely rely on your professional advisers and skip Chapter 6).

When You Can Give

Charitable donations can be made at any time that best meets your personal, tax, and other goals. The timing of a gift is considerably flexible. Even if a charitable gift won't be effective until some future date, it can still benefit the Society immediately by encouraging others to give and by giving assurance of future funding. Confirming a future gift today ensures that that gift will occur. Waiting to make the gift in the future, without creating a contractual arrangement today, will be far less likely to result in a donation. Contributions to fund the cure can be divided into four categories based on the timing of the donations. These time periods are important to understand because they affect the planning opportunities available to you and other prospective donors:

Inter-vivos Contributions. You can give gifts to the Society while you are alive. These are called inter-vivos gifts or lifetime contributions. The simplest and most obvious inter-vivos gift is for you to write out a check. But many other types of lifetime contributions are possible. You can make gifts of appreciated assets while you are alive. You can structure a charitable gift using a charitable remainder trust, charitable lead trust, or other techniques (all explained in later chapters). These more sophisticated techniques can enable you to accomplish goals that a mere cash contribution cannot, such as benefiting yourself or a loved one with MS, while still helping to fund the cure.

Testamentary Contributions. You can plan gifts that will only take effect on your death. These are called testamentary gifts or post-death contributions. The simplest and most obvious testamentary gift is for you to include a bequest to the Society in your will, revocable living trust (a lifetime trust in which the charitable beneficiary only obtains the gift on your death), or any other legal document taking effect on your death. There are many additional ways in which you can make a post-death gift, as described below.

✱ EXAMPLE: Jane Harrison is concerned that she faces a significant estate tax, but she is reluctant to engage in planning because of the uncertainty of future changes in the estate tax. Jane's goal is to benefit the Society and her heirs, but to preserve flexibility to modify her plan if significant new changes occur in the estate tax. She can always change her will to reflect modifications or changes in her overall plan. So, Jane bequeaths that portion of her estate that is not subject to federal estate tax ($2 million in 2007, but scheduled to increase) directly to her children. Jane makes a bequest of a significant portion of her remaining assets under her will in a manner that is structured as a charitable lead trust (CLT). This means that Jane's will bequeaths assets to a trust that will provide the Society with cash payments for 20 years; after that time, the remaining assets will benefit her designated heirs. Because they will receive $2 million on Jane's death, and the balance 20 years later, Jane views the deferral of the children's bequest positively as akin to a forced savings or retirement plan for them. The 20-year income interest (actually an annuity payment) to the Society could eliminate most estate tax on the bequest (see Chapters 3 through 6). Because this type of trust will only become effective on her death, it is referred to as a testamentary trust.

Although a gift made while you are alive will benefit the Society more quickly than a post-death gift, considering gifts made following death can open up opportunities for many new gifts and new donors under circumstances that gifts made during your lifetime cannot. For example, if you were diagnosed with MS and want to make a contribution to help fund the cure, you might be wary of dissipating current resources until you have a better handle on your post-diagnosis financial picture. However, you might be quite willing to make a testamentary commitment with the hopes of making additional gifts while you are alive when you feel comfortable doing so.

The following illustrates a sample clause you could include in your will to benefit the Society with an unrestricted gift:

✪ EXAMPLE: I direct my Executor to distribute and pay over to the National Multiple Sclerosis Society, with its principal offices in New York, New York, $25,000, for its general use and purposes.

Current Contributions. You can give a gift that takes effect immediately. These are called current gifts or contributions. The simplest and most obvious current gift is for you to write out a check. You can also donate property (e.g., appreciated stock) to the Society today as a current gift. Charitable remainder trusts are not current gifts, because the Society only receives the actual benefit at some future date. Current gifts help immediately to fund the cure.

Deferred Contributions. You can give a gift that takes effect only at some future date. These are called future or deferred gifts or contributions. The simplest and most obvious deferred gift is for you to include a bequest to the Society in your will. You could make a commitment to pay off a bequest over several years, which would be considered a deferred gift (e.g., pledge $10,000 as a total gift, to be paid $5,000/year, starting next year). You can make deferred gifts using any type of trust that will make a distribution to the Society at some future date. A charitable remainder trust takes effect in the future, and is an example of a trust that creates a deferred contribution. These more sophisticated techniques can enable you to accomplish goals that a mere cash contribution cannot, such as benefiting yourself or a loved one with MS while still helping to fund the cure. Deferred gifts are also referred to as planned gifts, because you have to plan their payment. Although dollars from deferred gifts cannot directly help fund the cure immediately, they can help immediately to encourage others to make contributions. Deferred gifts can also open many opportunities for gifts that could not be made on a current basis. Thus, deferred gifts, over time, can help the Society raise new additional dollars to help fund the cure. Deferred gifts enable the Society to plan future expenditures and programs.

Combination Contributions. You can make a contribution to the Society that meets all the above timing criteria. To help understand the relationship of the timing of gifts, bear in mind that all "current" or "present" gifts are lifetime gifts, but "future gifts" can be either lifetime or testamentary. Some gift plans can include elements of lifetime, testamentary, current, and deferred methods. Although this might sound complicated, it can actually be quite simple, and it allows you to provide tremendous benefit to the Society, including certainty that the organization can plan future expenditures (e.g., when budgeting for a particular program).

How Long Is Your Donation Effective: Perpetual Gifts

Annual gifts are the financial foundations of most charities. Annual gifts provide the funding, year to year, to continue essential programs and services, as well as to cover the administrative costs of operating most charities. But, although annual gifts are vital and clearly will contribute to funding the cure, each year professional staff or volunteers must again raise those same dollars to continue programs funded in the prior year. For those donors who are willing and able, there is a better way. And if you're willing, there are many creative ways to become "able" to do it in a better way. What is that better way? You could endow (make permanent) your annual contribution.

⚲   EXAMPLE: Jane Smith's daughter, Susan Smith, lives with the challenges of MS. When Jane first learned of her daughter's diagnosis, she made a donation of $5,000 to the Society. She has continued to make an annual $5,000 donation. Jane views this as just another way to show her daughter support and encouragement. Jane is in relative good health and just turned 70. Jane knows that, when she dies, her $5,000 annual donations will cease. For her daughter's sake, Jane would like to have her annual donations to the Society continue in the future, but she doesn't want to offend her son, who is less supportive of her daughter's situation. Jane decides against making a bequest in her will to the Society to perpetuate (endow) her annual gift because it will be so visible to her son. Jane fears doing so would only antagonize him, and thus lessen the likelihood of him ever stepping up to the plate to help his sister. Jane instead opts to purchase a life insurance policy to be owned by the Society and payable to the organization on her death. In this way, for an additional annual gift (i.e., Jane's $5,000 annual gift, which she will continue, and the cost of an annual insurance premium, which she will donate as well), Jane can ensure that her annual gift will continue forever.

Endowing your annual contribution is one of the most important and powerful steps you can take to help the Society fund the cure. However, some care must be taken in endowing your annual gift. How should you plan and structure the perpetuation of your annual gift? How can the Society practically administer an endowment that is to last for years? Many donors haven't really thought through the implications of a perpetual gift. For example, the famous Barnes Foundation was created in 1922, and now owns an art collection valued at approximately $6 billion. The original goal of the foundation was to maintain and display the art collection in a house in Marion, Pennsylvania. However, in 2004, a judge expanded the number of trustees for the foundation and authorized them to build a more traditional museum in downtown Philadelphia, because the foundation was no longer viable in its original structure. How do you plan a gift that will last in perpetuity in the manner that you, as donor, want without creating undue problems for the Society? Use a written gift document that addresses many of the potential options that might occur and addresses how your endowment should be handled if a particular option occurs:

- If you name a particular family member to designate how each year's contribution should be used, what if that family member can no longer serve in that capacity? Who is the successor? What if that successor dies? You must establish a workable protocol to make sure that decision-making positions are always staffed.

- Include a detailed alternative "Plan B" and even "Plan C," because over time a gift may become impractical, things change, and you'll never anticipate them all. Focus on flexibility.
- Provide a minimum amount which, if your fund declines in value to that level, the monies will be distributed and the fund terminated. Below some specified amount (which will vary depending on your objectives for the fund), it is simply not practical to expect a charity to administer the fund. Your goal is to help the Society find a cure, not waste scarce resources administering the small amount of dollars remaining in your depleted fund.

❂ EXAMPLE: Jane Smith purchased a life insurance policy on herself, to be owned by the Society and to benefit the organization. Jane and the Society signed a written agreement to establish the Susan Smith Research Fund. Jane has donated a significant sum each year to the Society and directed that it be used to fund research efforts that Jane believes, after consultation with expert investigators recommended by the Society, will best advance the development of medications to help certain bladder conditions that her daughter and tens of thousands of others with Primary Progressive MS have. Jane anticipates that, on her death, her daughter Susan will assume the responsibility for allocating the funds to be distributed. However, recognizing Susan's frailty, Jane names Susan's husband and several alternative persons to assume this responsibility. Hoping that this narrowly defined research and funding project will succeed, Jane provides in the written agreement with the Society that, if this narrow purpose is no longer practical or necessary, the person named in the agreement can allocate the funds for any other research or programming efforts of the organization. Finally, being practical about administrative burdens, Jane provides in the agreement that if the balance in her fund ever declines to $25,000 or less, all the remaining money will be donated outright to the Society for its general purposes, and the fund will be terminated.

Comprehensive Example of When and How You Can Give

The various times at which you can make a contribution can be illustrated using an example that will also show you how to tailor these different time periods to meet different objectives, as well as a few of the many options that might be available in such a plan. This example will be developed to illustrate the expansion of a simple donation into a more comprehensive and valuable donation that can achieve the goals of a particular donor while assuring that the Society receives vital support, including a perpetual endowment of the annual contribution.

✱ EXAMPLE 1: **Current, Inter-Vivos, Annual Gift:** Robert Smith is a regular contributor to the Society. Annually, he contributes $10,000 to fund services for his state's MS chapter to provide programming for those newly diagnosed with MS. He remembers well the emotional trauma his sister experienced when she was first diagnosed with MS. He also remembers the help, encouragement, and support her local Society chapter provided to her at that difficult time. Robert wanted to help expand those services, especially for those newly diagnosed who don't have the strong family support his sister had. So, his annual $10,000 gift is designated to fund programs for those newly diagnosed with MS living in his sister's state. The donation is a current gift, since he made a payment this year. This is an inter-vivos gift since, it is made while Robert is alive. The benefits to the local chapter from this gift are significant, because the chapter can fund the cost of an important program that would not have been expanded to the level it has without Robert's personal commitment, encouragement, and financial help. This is an important component in making a charitable gift: In many cases, the gift is not only the dollars that a particular donor gives, but the encouragement, ideas, and leadership to make a particular program happen. Robert, after sharing his sister's experience, had a personal interest in easing that particular situation for others.

✪ EXAMPLE 2: **Planned Gift:** Robert Smith could do more to ensure that his goals are met. The programs he funds must be budgeted and approved every year, based on whether his donation is received. Robert did not realize that originally, and he would prefer to give the local chapter the certainty of knowing that the annual gift will continue, so that they can plan accordingly in the future. Robert has always intended to fund this donation each year, so he gladly agreed to sign a pledge card committing to do so. Robert's gift has now become a planned gift, in that a plan exists to continue paying it. It is also now a deferred gift (as well as a current gift), since his pledge will be paid in future years. The advantage to the local Society chapter of knowing that the program will be funded for the foreseeable future is tremendous. Resources can be allocated appropriately, and uncertainty is removed. For Robert, knowing that this program will continue is a significant reward, well beyond the valuable income tax deduction he receives each year.

✪ EXAMPLE 3: **Simple Testamentary Bequest to Perpetuate Annual Gift:** Robert Smith could do more to ensure that his goals are met even further into the future. If Robert dies, his annual gifts will cease, and so might the additional program he has encouraged and supported financially. Although Robert never considered these risks, when approached by his sister, he was grateful when she pointed this out. Robert would like to ensure that, when he dies, his gifts to the Society will continue. How can his regular $10,000 annual contribution continue? Robert wants to endow his annual $10,000 gift to ensure that, even after his death, the Society will receive forever (in perpetuity) $10,000 each year to fund these activities (see the discussion of perpetual gifts below). Robert is concerned that if he doesn't perpetuate this particular annual gift, it might be difficult for the Society to replace this gift and the programming, which he feels is so important. Robert can include the language below in his will to ensure that the $10,000 pledged amount will be paid to the Society forever. Because this latter component of the gift is made under Robert's will, it is referred a testamentary gift. Because this contribution will only occur at some future date, it is also referred to as a future or deferred gift. Since this gift is planned (in contrast to his $10,000 annual check), it is also called a planned gift. Robert decides that, if he can bequeath $166,667 to the Society for this program, the program should receive adequate funding in all future years. He based his decision on the assumption that the bequest of $166,667 should reasonably be able to earn 6% and pay the $10,000 annual contribution forever.

▶ SAMPLE WILL CLAUSE

I, Robert Smith, direct my Executor to distribute and pay over to the National Multiple Sclerosis Society, with its principal offices in New York, New York (the Society), $166,667, and that a fund be established in my name, the income of which shall be used toward the funding of programming for those newly diagnosed with multiple sclerosis in the state of Wisconsin. I recognize that the need for this type of programming may change over time, and therefore authorize the Society to redirect the income from this fund to reasonable alternative purposes if it deems advisable. No interest shall be paid on this pledge. If the Society has been subject to a change in name, or merger into a successor organization serving substantially the same purposes, such organization shall be considered to exist and the gift and bequest above shall not lapse.

✪ EXAMPLE 4: **Ensuring That The Endowment of the Annual Gift Keeps Pace with Inflation:** Robert Smith consults his financial planner, who explains to him the impact of inflation on a perpetual gift and makes suggestions as to how Robert can better structure the bequest to ensure that his goals are carried out. The financial planner explains that, because of inflation, a fixed $10,000 gift per year will diminish in purchasing power over the years, possibly reaching a point at which, in terms of current dollars, the programs Robert wishes to perpetuate may not be able to be supported from the funds he plans to contribute. The financial planner recommends that several important changes be made to Robert's bequest. First, no more than 4% per year should be paid out of the fund Robert establishes. This should permit the principal amount to remain intact on an inflation-adjusted basis. Second, instead of paying a fixed dollar amount (such as 6% of the initial gift, as illustrated in the preceding example), a percentage of the fund should be paid each year. If the fund is $250,000 in its initial year, the 4% payment will be $10,000, as planned. If the fund grows to $260,000 in the second year, then 4% of $260,000, or $10,400 will be paid. This concept, Robert's financial planner explains, is referred to as a unit-trust payment. This will likely ensure that the programs Robert so cherishes will be able to continue in perpetuity despite the impact of inflation. This constitutes a true endowment. It requires a somewhat larger bequest initially, and a somewhat more complex payout, but will give far greater assurance of Robert's goals being achieved. If Robert wanted to quantify the likelihood of this revised endowment plan succeeding, he could have his financial planner simulate thousands of hypothetical investment/payment scenarios and actually determine the probability of achieving the goal of perpetual funding. While this might sound complex, many financial planners, wealth managers, and investment advisors are well equipped to perform this type of analysis and help plan perpetual gifts for donors like Robert.

▶ SAMPLE WILL CLAUSE

I, Robert, Smith, direct my Executor to distribute and pay over to the National Multiple Sclerosis Society, with its principal offices in New York, New York (the Society), $250,000 and that a fund be established in my name, the distributions of which shall be used toward the funding of programming for those newly diagnosed with multiple sclerosis in the state of Wisconsin. The distribution from this fund in each calendar year shall be Four Percent (4%) of the fair market value of this fund on January 1 of that calendar year (or, for the initial year, the fair market value of this fund on the first day of the receipt of assets by this fund). This distribution amount shall be payable once per year within Sixty (60) days of the valuation date. The distribution amount shall not be prorated for any partial year. I recognize that the need for this type of programming may change over time and therefore authorize the

Society to redirect the income from this fund to reasonable alternative purposes if it deems advisable. No interest shall be paid on this pledge. If the Society has been subject to a change in name, or merger into a successor organization serving substantially the same purposes, such organization shall be considered to exist and the gift and bequest above shall not lapse.

✪ EXAMPLE 4: **Starting to Fund a Perpetual Gift Today:** Robert Smith consults his accountant, who suggests that he begin to contribute some money this year to create the fund to endow his annual gift in perpetuity. Robert's accountant explains that Robert can contribute appreciated stock to the Society to start the fund and get great current income tax benefits (see Chapter 6). Robert's accountant also explains that, although Robert currently faces a significant estate tax, it is possible that if the estate tax exclusion (the amount everyone can give away without any federal estate tax) is increased significantly, Robert's estate may not realize any estate tax benefit from the charitable contribution to the Society, so he might be better off making contributions while alive to obtain an income tax deduction. So, Robert will establish the fund today with the Society, with a modest initial contribution. Each year, when Robert meets with his accountant to discuss year-end tax planning, they'll review Robert's portfolio and harvest stocks with large taxable gains to donate to Robert's fund. The accountant will coordinate the impact of this on Robert's investment allocation with Robert's financial planner. To implement this plan, one additional change must be made to Robert's will because now Robert's estate only needs to donate to his fund the shortfall between the $250,000 pledge to perpetually endow his annual gift and the actual dollars donated to this fund in prior years. This approach is necessary to build flexibility into Robert's will, because it is uncertain when he will die and how much money will be in his fund from inter-vivos donations (gifts while he is alive). Although this planning adds a bit more complexity, it is the exact type of planning most high-income or high–net worth donors should consider. When you coordinate your charitable planning, income and estate tax planning, financial planning, and all of your advisers are involved in this process, significant benefits can be realized.

▶ SAMPLE WILL CLAUSE

I, Robert Smith, direct my Executor to distribute and pay over to the National Multiple Sclerosis Society, with its principal offices in New York, New York (the Society), the amount necessary so that the "Robert Smith Fund" established November 22, 2007, has a balance as of the date of my death not less than $250,000 (inclusive of all prior donations to such fund, income accumulated on less income paid out of such a fund prior to my death, and this *bequest under my Last Will and Testament). I direct that this fund make distributions which shall be used toward the funding of programming for those newly diagnosed with multiple sclerosis in the state of Wisconsin. The distribution from this fund in each calendar year shall be Four Percent (4%) of the fair market value of this fund on January 1 of that calendar year (or, for the year of my death, the fair market value of this fund on the first day after the receipt of assets distributed to this fund by my estate). This distribution amount shall be payable once per year within Sixty (60) days of the valuation date. The distribution amount shall not be prorated for any partial year. I recognize that the need for this type of programming may change over time and therefore authorize the Society to redirect the income from this fund to reasonable alternative purposes if it deems advisable. No interest shall be paid on this pledge. If the Society has been subject to a change in name, or merger into a successor organization serving substantially the same purposes, such organization shall be considered to exist and the gift and bequest above shall not lapse.*

What You Can Give

Too many donors and prospective donors believe the only choice of contributions is cash, check, or credit card. Although every charity welcomes these types of cash donations, the opportunities to contribute are far broader. By carefully picking which assets you gift to help fund the cure, you can maximize income and possibly other tax benefits, and accomplish a host of personal goals as well. Detailed examples and discussions of each of the following items you can donate (as well as other items), will be presented in Chapter 4.

Cash Contributions: Cash contributions, whether in the form of cash, a check, or a credit card payment are simple to make (although as illustrated earlier and throughout this book, even cash donations can take many sophisticated forms).

Tangible Property Contributions: You can donate tangible personal property, such as art, jewelry, or other property to a charity. However, these types of donations raise practical, tax, and other issues. If you donate a grand piano, how will it be transported? Who will bear the cost of transport? Will it be used in an MS Center providing programming services, or will it simply be sold? There are a number of tough restrictions on the donation of tangible property such as artwork. The tax ramifications could be significant (see Chapter 6).

Intangible Property Contributions: Stocks, bonds, life insurance policies, and other intangible assets (contractual rights, in contrast to tangible property such as art or furniture) can also be donated. Some beneficial ways to do this have been illustrated earlier in this chapter.

Real Property Contributions: Real estate can often be donated to a charity. This can provide tremendous tax and other benefits. You can make gifts of interests in your home, commercial real estate, and more (see Chapter 4).

Service Contributions: You may not have the financial wherewithal to contribute, but you always have a very important asset to contribute—yourself. Giving of your time, energy, and heart has and always will be the most important and inspirational contribution. It's far easier to write out a check than to donate your time to help an individual or group of people living with the challenges of MS, or to see a project from its initial vision to reality. In fact, a tremendous way to contribute when you don't have the financial resources personally is to inspire and educate other potential donors who have the financial wherewithal to make significant financial donations, like those described in this book. Many wealthy prospective donors have a connection to MS and a desire to help, but simply are not aware of the many options for gifting, especially how to give while simultaneously helping themselves or their loved ones.

Who Can Give

Who can make a charitable contribution? Charitable gifts can be made by a number of different people or entities as a result of your efforts and planning. It can be far more flexible than just you writing out a check. By considering the various people and entities that can make donations for you, or because of your efforts, you can realize a host of additional benefits.

Donor with MS: Charitable gifts can be made directly by you, the donor. Your personal experiences with MS give you a unique perspective on how you might want to help the Society's research efforts.

Family and Friends of Someone with MS: While someone with MS may not be in a position to make significant gifts because of the detrimental impact MS has had on their earnings and savings, loved ones may be in a position to give. These gifts can be used in many ways to directly (e.g., charitable lead trust) or indirectly (the Society succeeds in finding a cure) benefit the family member or friend with MS.

Compassionate Donor: Some donors have no direct family or friends affected by MS but have become aware of the physical, cognitive, social, and financial consequences MS can bring and, out of sheer benevolence, want to help fund the cure. There are a multitude of ways this can be done, as discussed in Chapters 3 through 6, and many of these methods can be planned to generate income, gift, estate, or other tax benefits.

Agent: Every adult should sign a basic estate planning document called a durable (remains effective even if you are disabled) power of attorney. This document authorizes a person you name, your "agent" to handle your financial and legal affairs if you cannot do so yourself. When any prospective donor signs a power of attorney, the agent named in the power of attorney can be authorized to make charitable contributions on the donor's behalf. However, for this to be possible, the power of attorney legal document should expressly give the agent authority to make charitable contributions and indicate the scope of that authority. For example, the power could authorize the donor's agent to make gifts to the Society in amounts not in excess of the maximum contributions made to the organization in any one of the three years preceding the donor's disability. If you have a specific charitable plan in place that requires actions in future years (e.g., you pledge $50,000 to be paid $10,000/year starting two years from now), your power of attorney should expressly authorize your agent to carry out your plan. If it doesn't, then in the event of your disability, your plan may never be implemented.

If you have MS, you should have a comprehensive durable power of attorney that authorizes a named agent and several successors to handle a wide range of financial and legal matters for you. If you have a loved one with MS, you should be certain that you too have a durable power of attorney and that it expressly authorizes your agent to make payments for the care of your loved ones. If not, your agent may not be able to do so.

Trustee: The trustee under your revocable living trust could make charitable gifts. But, similar to the issues noted in the context of an agent under your power of attorney, the trustee under your trust should expressly be authorized to make charitable gifts. If not, a question may arise as to whether the trustee is authorized to do so. If you create a charitable trust, the trustees will be authorized to make charitable gifts based on the terms of that trust.

> ✪ EXAMPLE: You establish a charitable remainder trust (CRT). A CRT is a special trust that requires a payment be made periodically, perhaps annually, to you for a set number of years or life. This payment can be made to you and your spouse (or in some instances, other beneficiaries). So, the trustee of the CRT could be required by the terms of the trust document to pay you and your husband a 7% annuity every year for your joint lives. If you contribute $1 million to this CRT, the trustee must pay $70,000 each year until the last of you dies. At that time, after any final payment due on the $70,000 annual payments, the balance of the trust must be distributed to the Society as the charitable beneficiary. Your trustee is not only authorized, she is required, to make this charitable distribution.

Designated Heirs: If you have a loved one living with MS, the uncertainty MS creates might in part be offset by empowering that loved one to allocate the charitable gifts you make to the Society to fund projects they deem important. This element of control and involvement can itself be an important benefit you can bestow. You might do this in one of several ways:

- You could donate money or property to the Society and have these monies held in a separate fund under your name, to be used to fund various research or other projects designated by your loved one in future years.

  ❁ EXAMPLE: Dorothy Harrington, as the donor, establishes a $100,000 charitable fund with the Society. Dorothy and the Society enter into a written agreement governing the terms of how the fund will be used. The agreement provides that Dorothy's niece, Jennifer, who lives with MS, will direct the distribution of charitable contributions to the Society each year.

- A common charitable planning technique is for donors to establish donor-advised funds. In a typical donor-advised fund arrangement, you could donate appreciated stock before the end of the year to a major public charity and obtain a current income tax deduction without designating the specific charities to receive contributions. In later years, you can then designate qualified charities, and your donor-advised fund could distribute money to the named charity, such as the Society.

- If you have sufficient resources and charitable intent, you could establish a private foundation. Your heirs could be designated as having authority on behalf of the foundation to make determinations concerning charitable distributions.

Business: Businesses can also make charitable contributions. This can range from a large employer matching employee donations, to gifts of inventory (e.g., a supermarket donates snacks for use by participants in an MS Walk), to corporate sponsorships or even donations of the business itself.

Chapter Summary

Charitable giving can be far more flexible and dynamic than just writing out a check. You can give donations that are effective at many different times, using a wide range of assets that can last for various durations and can even be directed by many different people. Your awareness of these options will help open the door for you to identify many different ways that you, or other prospective donors you know, might be able to donate to the Society while achieving important personal and tax goals, and thus help to fund the cure.

CHAPTER THREE

HELPING PEOPLE YOU CARE ABOUT THROUGH CHARITABLE GIVING

PEOPLE OR CAUSES YOU CARE ABOUT are usually at the heart (literally) of most charitable giving. Because the tax rate is nowhere near 100%, you are always better off keeping your money or assets than giving them to charity. So, even though tax breaks are important, you give to help a cause, goal, or person you are concerned about. This chapter explores how you can use charitable giving to benefit someone you care about and also benefit the National Multiple Sclerosis Society (the Society). The person might be yourself, a loved one or friend affected by MS, or simply someone you want to benefit or protect.

Yourself

If you're living with the challenges of MS, a carefully crafted charitable plan can help you as well as the Society. Charitable giving can benefit you in a host of ways. Consider the following:

First, Protect Yourself: The most important, and obvious, indirect benefit is that your charitable efforts help the Society underwrite the costs of research projects that may just lead to discoveries of new therapies that will help you. You might wish, in light of the financial uncertainty of MS, to simply harvest (select) your most highly appreciated investment positions each year and donate a portion of these to the Society. This gives you the ultimate flexibility to determine what is appropriate to contribute each year, provides for substantial income tax benefits (see Chapter 6 for more details), and will give you the feeling of having taken action. Sometimes the simplest techniques are the most appropriate. In the meantime, the efforts and expenditures you might have put into more sophisticated charitable planning (such as those described below) can be channeled into ensuring that your assets are optimally organized and invested and your estate planning documents revised to best protect you against the potential trajectory your disease may take. When these essential steps are completed, and you've had a few years to assimilate the consequences of your diagnosis, you can then revisit more comprehensive charitable planning.

Donate Appreciated Stocks: If you sell appreciated securities, you will generally pay a capital gains tax. You then have to invest and manage the proceeds. Instead, however, you could give your appreciated securities to the Society in exchange for a gift annuity. This arrangement gives you a charitable contribution deduction (which will vary based on your age), and you will be entitled to receive an annuity for the rest of your life. This not only provides an income tax benefit, but it also eliminates your need to manage the assets. If you are dealing with the demands and stresses of life with MS, having a portion of your portfolio converted to an annuity might be appropriate for you. But, unlike a commercial annuity, a gift annuity with the Society has the important additional benefit of knowing that you will be supporting the organization's projects. You must be cautious about how much you commit to gift annuities, because you cannot access the principal in the event of an emergency.

Consider a CRT: If you operate your own business or manage real estate property, and it is getting more difficult for you as your disease progresses, or you simply feel you need to reduce the stress that managing a business or property causes, donate the business or the real estate to a charitable remainder trust (CRT). This trust may then sell the asset (without being assessed a capital gains tax) and reinvest the proceeds, which could pay you a monthly annuity for life. This annuity may cover a significant portion or all of your living expenses. As with gift annuities, you must be cautious about how much you commit to a CRT, because you cannot access the principal in the event of an emergency. Thus, in most CRT plans, a portion of the asset may be sold and a portion contributed to a CRT. On your death, the money remaining in the CRT will be given to the Society. See Chapters 4 through 6 for a more detailed discussion.

Implement a Revocable Living Trust: For anyone living with MS, establishing a revocable living trust to manage your assets through the difficulties of an exacerbation or in the event of a more significant permanent disability is an important estate, financial, and personal planning step. If you do set up a trust to provide for the management of your assets, you should consider permitting some amount of charitable donations by your trustees, including the possible purchase of gift annuities from the Society if appropriate. This is important, because if contributions and even gift annuities aren't addressed specifically, your trustee may be precluded from taking these steps, or may be so concerned about violating his fiduciary duties as trustee that he might refrain from doing so even if not absolutely prohibited by law.

Spouse

Protecting Your Spouse and Benefiting the Society

If your spouse has MS, many planning opportunities are available that use charitable giving to benefit and protect your spouse, while also benefiting the Society. One of the key steps to protecting your spouse is the use of trusts to provide for the management of assets and other assistance if your spouse's condition warrants such help. Trusts are legal arrangements (contracts) in which assets are owned and managed by a trustee for the benefit of beneficiaries, such as your spouse. Trusts create a safety net that can enable your spouse to stay in complete control, but have other persons as trustees or successor trustees poised to assist, if and when necessary. Using creative charitable planning, trusts can be created in forms that protect your spouse, save estate tax, obtain charitable contribution tax benefits, and benefit the Society.

In many instances, you may only wish to consummate a charitable gift following the continued personal use of the property by your spouse. While you could simply wait and make the contribution at a future date, structuring the gift now locks in the protection, planning results, and, in some instances, may qualify for a current income tax charitable deduction. The contribution that occurs after a time of personal use is referred to as a remainder interest, since it remains after the period of personal use. If your spouse is given the right to live in your home for life and, on his death, the home is given to the Society, the organization is said to have a remainder interest in the house.

Spouse Who Is Not a Citizen of the United States

Special rules apply if your spouse is not a citizen of the United States. In those cases, a special type of trust, a qualified domestic trust (QDOT), must be used to qualify for the gift or estate tax marital deduction. The amount of gifts that can be made in any year without a gift tax cost are also limited. If your spouse is not a citizen, you'll need to review these special rules with your tax adviser.

Charitable Remainder Trust to Benefit a Spouse

The charitable remainder trust (CRT) technique was introduced briefly in Chapter 2. The typical or "plain vanilla" use of a CRT is for you to donate appreciated property to the CRT, which sells the property without incurring capital gains; you receive an income tax charitable contribution deduction, and the CRT pays you an annual annuity for life. This plain vanilla CRT plan can be modified in different ways so that you can achieve the goal of protecting a spouse with MS and assuring him a cash flow for life, free of any responsibility to manage the assets. Each variation discussed below can also help you accomplish important tax saving and charitable goals. In many cases, a combination of these techniques may provide the best result. In almost all situations, these techniques must be part of an overall estate and financial plan that addresses all your and your spouse's needs and goals, and these techniques will only be used for a portion of your wealth.

Marital Gift Followed by Spousal CRT: If you have assets, such as appreciated growth stock mutual funds, you can gift them to your spouse. Your spouse can then establish a CRT for his or her benefit, and contribute the appreciated mutual funds to the CRT. The CRT can continue the current investments as long as necessary, then, at the appropriate time, sell the growth mutual funds and reinvest the proceeds, free of any capital gains tax, into income-oriented funds. The income from the CRT's revised asset allocation strategy can be used to pay your spouse an annuity for life. He or she won't have to manage the assets and will be free from those pressures. An income tax charitable contribution deduction could be realized on your joint income tax return when the CRT is initially formed and the mutual funds contributed. When the CRT sells the mutual funds, no capital gains tax should apply. Your spouse can have an annuity payment made quarterly for the rest of his or her life. On his or her death, the Society will receive the remaining assets held in the CRT. But the Society will realize intangible benefits from the date the CRT is initially formed in that it will be able to reflect the commitment in its efforts to engage other donors.

Create a Joint Spousal CRT: Instead of giving assets to your spouse to fund a trust for him or her only, you might feel that you need some of the income (really cash flow in the form of an annuity payment) for your future expenses (e.g., your retirement). So, instead of having just your spouse set up the CRT, you can set up a CRT that pays a joint annuity payment to both of you for life. This will assure you that, if your spouse dies before you, you will continue to receive an annuity payment for the remainder of your life. Thus, the annuity payment from the CRT to you and your spouse will continue for the longer of your life or the life of your spouse. There will be no estate tax on either your death or the death of your spouse. On your death, your estate will qualify for both a charitable contribution deduction and an estate tax marital deduction. This ensures that no tax is applied as a result of any interest you had in the CRT on death.

An illustration of a CRT will help you understand how you can benefit your spouse and the Society using a CRT.

> ✪ EXAMPLE: Adam Jones wants to provide for the protection of his wife, Cindy, who lives with MS. Adam contemplates donating $1 million of stock that he has held for many years and has appreciated substantially over its $150,000 purchase price (tax basis). Because Adam has already engaged in considerable estate planning to benefit their children, he would like to benefit the Society following his and Cindy's deaths. Adam is hopeful that setting up this type of future benefit for the Society will encourage others to make major current and deferred gifts, thereby hastening the research that will hopefully help his wife. Adam decides to establish an inter-vivos (while he is alive) CRT for both himself and Cindy. Both Adam and Cindy will obtain current interests in the CRT. A current income tax deduction will be permitted, based on the present value of the future interest the Society

will receive. A deduction is permitted because the rights of the Society are fixed in a manner that conforms to the tax law requirements for a current deduction. A specified payout must occur in each year (or more frequent period if you wish to provide for it in the trust). No additional payments may be made to Adam or Cindy, other than those fixed in the CRT document when it is established. Properly structured, this will also qualify for a gift tax marital deduction (since Adam is making a gift to Cindy through the annuity payments she will receive for her life). However, should Cindy face an emergency, the trustees cannot distribute the principal of the trust to her, so Adam has made sure other resources are available to her in the event of an emergency. On the death of the last of Adam and Cindy, the principal remaining in the trust is to be distributed to the Society to establish a research grant in their memory. The Society is a *remainder beneficiary* of the CRT.

Combining Charitable and Marital Planning

Although the tax benefits of a CRT are substantial, there is a major drawback you must consider, especially if your spouse has MS. Once assets are contributed to the CRT, you cannot access the principal. The only right you and your spouse have is to receive the annuity payments as planned for in the trust agreement that creates the CRT. Thus, even if one of the CRT approaches described here is great for some of your wealth, it is unlikely to be appropriate for all your assets. Another approach is to take advantage of both the charitable contribution deduction and the marital deduction. You could establish a commonly used *marital trust* to protect your spouse in your will. This trust can protect your spouse by providing professional management of the assets in the trust, trustees who can pay bills and handle other matters for your spouse if necessary, protection from lawsuits and claims, and other benefits. If your will establishes this commonly used trust for your spouse, no estate tax will be applicable upon your death. If your spouse is a United States citizen, the most commonly used trust of this nature is called a qualified terminable interest property or "QTIP" trust. The significant advantage of this trust over the CRT is that, in an emergency, the trustees can invade the principal of the trust and use any or all of it for the care of your spouse. Then, following the death of your spouse, whatever assets remain in the QTIP trust can be contributed to the Society. In tax parlance, the Society is the *remainder beneficiary* of this trust. While this approach is simpler and more flexible than the CRT, no income tax deduction is available with a QTIP with a charitable remainder, as there would be when a charitable remainder trust is used with you and your spouse named as income beneficiaries. In many cases, a combination of the techniques may present the best approach to protecting your spouse.

The following example illustrates how you, as a prospective donor, can accomplish the important personal goals of protecting your spouse who has MS and simultaneously creating a charitable plan to benefit the Society and the MS community:

✪ EXAMPLE: Cindy Jones' husband Sam has primary progressive MS. Cindy wants to provide protection for Sam for his life but, on his demise, Cindy wants to benefit the Society. Cindy establishes a inter-vivos (while she is alive) marital trust (QTIP) for her husband, Sam. Sam has a current interest in the trust. No current income tax deduction is permitted for the future interest the Society will receive after Sam's death. No deduction is permitted, because the rights of the Society as the charity are not fixed in a manner that conforms to the tax law requirements for a current deduction. To protect Sam, the trust may pay any necessary amounts of the trust principal (assets) to Sam, or for his benefit, during Sam's lifetime. A trust company is named as co-trustee with Sam. This assures Sam's involvement in his own trust, and assures that, if he can no longer fully participate in the management of the trust, a bank will provide for whatever financial and other services he needs. Properly structured, this trust will qualify for a gift tax marital deduction when Cindy establishes it. During Sam's lifetime, all income must be distributed at least annually. In addition, should Sam face an emergency, the trustees may distribute principal to him. On Sam's demise, the principal remaining in the trust is to be distributed to the Society, the remainder beneficiary. No current charitable contribution deduction will apply. However, upon Sam's death, although the value of the entire trust will be included in his taxable estate, an equal and offsetting charitable contribution deduction will apply.

Child

If you have a child diagnosed with MS, a host of steps are available for you to take to protect your child. Each of these steps might also be tailored to have a charitable connection. The following discussion reviews a few of the many possibilities based on some of the estate planning documents you might use in your own planning.

Power of Attorney

This common estate planning document designates a person (agent) to manage your financial, legal, and other affairs if you cannot do so. The historical development of the power of attorney is such that, if you have a child over the age of majority that you are not obligated by law to support, your agent cannot expend funds for that child. If your child has a severe course of MS, this could be financially devastating. So, it is vital that specific provisions be incorporated into your power of attorney that not only permit your agent to provide financial support to your child, but direct him to do so. Any gifts in excess of the annual gift tax exclusion ($12,000 in 2007, but the amount is inflation indexed) will be subject to tax. Your agent can make direct payments for medical or tuition expenses without limit and without gift tax consequences. While you are tailoring your power of attorney to address assisting your child, give some consideration to having your lawyer modify the gift provisions to include the right to make charitable gifts to the Society.

Revocable Living Trust

Many people use revocable living trusts to avoid probate, although a far more important use is to manage assets during illness or disability. If you have a revocable living trust as part of your estate plan, be sure to have your attorney make modifications similar to those described above for a power of attorney so that distributions (gifts) can be made to your child and the Society.

Will

Your will should probably include a trust to protect your child/beneficiary who is living with MS. The trust can provide for the management of assets in the event your child has reached a point at which he or she cannot easily manage his or her own financial affairs. Whether the situation is due to cognitive or physical impairments caused by MS, and whether this protection is required now or possibly at some time in the future, a trust tailored to protect your child while maintaining his or her involvement and dignity (perhaps as a co-trustee) is often the ideal solution. You'll have to address with the attorney drafting your will whether or not the trust should be a special needs trust (often referred to by its initials, SNT), depending on your child's financial and health condition. As with all estate planning documents, your will can provide a wonderful way to tailor a charitable bequest.

✱ EXAMPLE: Jim Johnson has two adult children, a son Thomas, and a daughter Sandy, who is in her thirties and has secondary progressive MS. Although Jim would have preferred to leave assets equally to his two children on his death, given the uncertainty about the progression of Sandy's MS, Jim is not sure this is fair. Some of the new grading systems being developed leave Jim cautiously optimistic that Sandy's MS won't progress to a level that will require him to distribute his estate unequally. But the predictive mechanisms based on disability and duration of the disease are relatively new, and he is concerned about how much reliance to place on them. After reviewing the matter with the family, Jim opts for the following disposition scheme in his will: 55% to Sandy, 40% to Thomas, and 5% to the Society. When Jim discusses this plan with his attorney, a couple of important issues are raised. While the likelihood exists that Sandy will need more financial assistance, that really cannot be known for certain, because the progression of her disease is unknown and new therapies are being developed. Just as importantly, Jim's attorney points out that there is no certainty that Thomas will not face some type of financial, health, or other adversity during his lifetime. Finally, Jim's attorney explains that, if a percentage of his estate is left to charity, the will and financial reporting must be submitted to the state's attorney general's office to comply with state law. Further, the attorney points out the valuation issues that can arise if a percentage of an estate is left to charity. Jim anticipates that the family vacation home in the country will be kept by both Thomas and Sandy for them and their children to use. For estate tax purposes, the children have the incentive to value the house as low as possible to minimize tax costs. However, the Society, as an independent charity, is obligated to ensure that fair market values are used. This disparity in goals could create some friction. The combination of these and other issues, the attorney explains, makes a donation of a percentage of the estate potentially problematic in Jim's particular situation. So, Jim settles on the following dispositive scheme: A fixed dollar bequest of $500,000 in his will to the Society, to be used to develop programming and facilities in the local Society chapter in which Sandy has been active. The remaining estate is divided into three components, 40% to each of Thomas and Sandy, in a separate trust designed to meet the specific needs of each child. The remaining 20% of the estate is distributed to a "pot" trust, which can benefit any child or grandchild based on need. That will enable Jim to distribute his estate in equal portions, but also ensure that if Sandy, or even Thomas, have more demanding issues, funds can be distributed to address those issues. The children and the Society all benefit from this revised plan.

Insurance Trust

A common estate planning tool is to establish a trust that purchases insurance on your life. The advantage of this approach is that the proceeds of the insurance will not be taxed in your estate on death, the cash value will be protected from your claimants, and the proceeds will be protected from claimants of your heirs. For families with a child with MS, an insurance trust can be used as a means of providing extra protection for that child.

> ✪ EXAMPLE: Janice Gordon has three children, two daughters and a son, Phillip, who has MS. Janice is adamant that her will bequeath assets equally, because she does not want to create any animosity or jealously among the children. Janice is especially concerned about keeping the peace, because her daughters have been wonderfully supportive and helpful of her son. However, Janice realistically understands that Phillip cannot work more than a limited amount and that, although his training as a CPA would have provided him a good living, the fatigue and cognitive problems caused by MS have limited his ability to maintain what Janice believes is an adequate lifestyle. So, Janice's will simply leaves all assets to her children equally. Janice establishes an irrevocable (cannot be changed) life insurance trust (sometimes referred to by its initials, ILIT) that purchases a $2 million universal policy on her life. This trust is

designed to help support and supplement Phillip. If Phillip marries and has children, on Phillip's death, the funds in the trust will be distributed to his children. Janice feels this is important, because Phillip does not have the capacity to earn a livelihood to support his children, and may not obtain life insurance because of his MS. If Phillip dies without children, the Society is named as the beneficiary of the remaining insurance proceeds. Janice believes that, for all the assistance that the Society has provided to her son, this would be a good way to acknowledge the organization and help others who also face the challenges of living with MS.

Charitable Lead Trust

A charitable lead trust (CLT) is designed to benefit charity and, at the same time, provide a future gift (inheritance) to your child at a substantially reduced gift (estate) tax cost. When you set up a CLT, the Society receives the income (actually an annuity payment) for a number of years that you agree to (the longer the number of years, the greater the tax break); thereafter, the assets in the trust will be distributed to your child. This is a great mechanism to benefit the Society, protect your child, and achieve tremendous tax savings. More details on this technique are explained in later chapters.

✪ EXAMPLE: Sally Stone, a widow, has a substantial estate. Her son and only heir, David, is age 40 and has MS. He continues to work and is self supporting. Sally wants to reduce both the potentially substantial estate tax she faces, while ensuring her son's financial future. Sally establishes a charitable lead annuity trust (CLAT) for her son. Sally has her attorney prepare a trust agreement, obtain a tax identification number, and the trustee sets up an account with the wealth management firm Sally has used for many years. Sally then donates $1 million dollars to the CLAT. The Society will receive $60,000 per year for the next 25 years. Sally directs that this be used to address vision problems caused by MS, so long as the Society deems a need for such research. She does not receive an income tax charitable contribution deduction. Assume that Sally has made prior gifts totaling $800,000 to her heirs, using up $800,000 of the $1 million gift tax exclusion available (the amount any taxpayer can gift without paying a gift tax). However, the $1 million gift could generate nearly $400,000 in gift tax cost [($1 million gift − $200,000 remaining exclusion) × 50% assumed tax rate]. However, because of the annuity payment of $60,000/year for 25 years, the value of the eventual gift to her son David is reduced to only about $200,000, and no gift tax will be payable on the transfer. From a personal perspective, not only has Sally provided substantial benefit to the Society, but she has provided a retirement plan for her son to ensure his financial security into old age. In 25 years, when David reaches age 65, the CLAT will end, and he will receive a distribution of the trust assets. Sally's wealth manager believes that it is reasonable for her to realize a 7.5% return on the CLAT portfolio, given the 25-year time horizon. As such, her son David will receive, not the original $1 million she gave to the CLAT, but in excess of $2 million when the trust terminates. Sally is confident that this amount will more than adequately fund her son's retirement years. If the CLAT is structured as what is referred to as a "grantor trust" (all CLAT income is taxed to Sally), then she would qualify for an income tax deduction each year. Most CLATs are not structured in this manner. Thus, in most instances, no income tax deduction is ever received. However, the gift tax consequence of the future gift to David can be reduced to nearly zero.

Charitable Remainder Trust

A charitable remainder trust (CRT) is almost exclusively thought of as a tax planning technique to benefit you, as the donor, and your spouse, if you are married. However, the CRT technique can be used to benefit a child as well, although there will be a gift tax consequence to this use. You'll have to be sure your estate planner structures the trust so that at least 10% of the initial value of the property you donate to the CRT will benefit the Society. This is necessary so that the trust will meet tax law requirements for you to obtain a contribution deduction. If you merely name your children (or perhaps just a child living with MS) as a beneficiary, a gift tax may be due on the formation of the trust. This gift tax consequence can be avoided if you retain in your will the right to terminate the children's interests under the CRT. This step, however, will cause the value of the CRT assets to be included in your estate at death. If you don't have a spouse, or if your spouse's life expectancy is limited, perhaps because of complications of his MS, this technique could be particularly useful. Depending on how the calculations play out, your heirs could actually receive a better economic arrangement using this approach than had you simply sold an appreciated asset, paid capital gains tax, and retained the proceeds to be included in your taxable estate. This is a complex technique that will require coordinated planning by your accountant, estate planner, and investment manager.

You can take several steps to protect a child with MS and in many cases weave in provisions to benefit the Society. These examples only illustrate a few of the myriad of planning possibilities, such as deferred gift annuities with income payable to the child in the future.

Grandchild

The financial planning for a grandchild with MS is similar to planning for a child with MS, with some exceptions. The most significant tax exception, and one that can have a tremendous impact on planning, is that gifts to grandchildren face severe restrictions if they are to avoid the generation-skipping transfer (GST) tax. This tax can be almost confiscatory in nature and must be carefully addressed by your estate planning attorney and accountant in any planning you undertake. The GST tax applies to transfers you make to "skip persons." In layman's terms, this includes grandchildren, trusts that only have grandchildren as beneficiaries, and other persons that are brought within the definition of "skip persons." Let's look at the same planning ideas discussed for your child with MS above, and see how they differ if you are endeavoring to assist a grandchild.

Power of Attorney

As explained earlier, your power designates a person (agent) to manage your financial, legal, and other affairs if you cannot do so. Your agent cannot spend money or make gifts for a grandchild unless you specifically authorize it. This contrasts with payments for a minor child, which your agent might be able to make without an express authorization. This may be the case because your state's laws may make it your legal obligation to support your minor children, so your agent would have the authority to make the necessary payments. Thus, for a grandchild with MS it's even more important that you're clear as to what your agent can spend. You could authorize gifts to grandchildren, but any gifts in excess of the annual gift tax exclusion ($12,000 in 2007, but the amount is inflation indexed) will have a gift and possibly a GST tax consequence as well. Direct payments for tuition and medical expenses can be made without any gift tax or GST tax consequences, if you authorize your agent to make them. For a grandchild, the direct payment of medical expenses by your agent could be a tremendous help to the grandchild, and a significant gift tax break for your estate. You should also address the issue of equality of gifts and other distributions in the document. Do you care if one grandchild receives more than another? Also, consider authorizing your agent to make charitable contributions to the Society.

Will

Your will should probably include a trust to protect your grandchild/beneficiary who is living with MS. The trust can provide for the management of assets in the event your grandchild reaches a point at which he or she cannot easily manage his or her own financial affairs, similar to the decisions discussed earlier concerning a child. You'll have to address with the attorney drafting your will whether the trust should be a special needs trust, depending on your grandchild's financial and health condition. This decision could be much more difficult to make for a grandchild, given their younger age and perhaps greater uncertainty as to the future progression of their MS. A significant difference in planning for a grandchild, as contrasted to a child, is the potential for GST tax. If total bequests to grandchildren exceed the GST exemption available to you ($2 million in 2007, but future increases or decreases are uncertain), your estate could face a substantial GST tax. If you are married, you and your spouse can each make bequests to a grandchild (or other *skip person*) for a total of $4 million. Thus, your will is likely to be more complex in that your estate planner will draft it so that the maximum bequests to grandchildren and trusts for grandchildren won't exceed the maximum GST exemption to which you are entitled. In many cases, the ability to make distributions for tuition and medical expenses can add some flexibility to provide for a grandchild with MS without unduly complicating your estate plan.

> ✪ EXAMPLE: Joe and Maria Davis have two adult children and four grandchildren, one of whom, Jerry, was recently diagnosed with MS. At this stage, they are not certain what Jerry's needs will be. The Davises also want to fund a gift to the Society to support publications to help young adults, especially those recently diagnosed. After reviewing various complex planning options with their attorney, the Davises opt for a fairly standard estate plan. On the death of the first of Joe or Maria, the maximum assets will be distributed to a by-pass trust, with the balance to a marital trust (QTIP designed to qualify for the unlimited estate tax marital deduction). The by-pass trust is designed to benefit the surviving spouse, but ensure that those assets are not included

in the estate of the surviving spouse. Under current law, $2 million can be contributed to such a trust (this amount may increase or decrease in future years). To provide flexibility, the trustee of the by-pass trust is authorized to make distributions to any of Joe and Maria's children but, to avoid GST issues, grandchildren are excluded from this general distribution provision. In addition, the Davises added the right for a trustee to distribute any monies directly to those providing medical or education benefits to Jerry, since such distributions won't trigger GST issues. The right to make distributions to Jerry's parents, as well as direct medical and education distributions, will provide flexibility and a safety net for Jerry. Rather than complicate their estate plan with charitable deductions, and especially in light of their desire to fund programs for young adults with MS now, the Davises simply make a cash gift to the Society.

Insurance Trust

The use of a life insurance trust (ILIT) to benefit a child with MS was discussed earlier. When the goal is to benefit a grandchild, the tax issues are more complex. Your advisors will help you address these issues. For example, the GST tax should also be considered. In many such situations, it will not be possible to qualify gifts to the insurance trust for the annual GST gift tax exemption, so your accountant will have to file a gift tax return each year to allocate GST exemption. Don't worry about these technicalities—your accountant will be equipped to address them for you. The next example will illustrate the planning, not the technicalities.

✪ EXAMPLE: Jeff and Susan Smith have three children, and two grandchildren, including a granddaughter Jane, who has MS. Jeff and Susan have their estate planner prepare an insurance trust primarily to benefit Jane. They have the trust purchase a $1 million survivorship (also called second-to-die) policy. This policy only pays when the last of Jeff and Susan dies. It is substantially cheaper than buying a policy on only one of their lives. Importantly, while either of Jeff or Susan are alive, they are confident that they can provide any extra help Jane needs. They are really only worried about providing for Jane after their deaths, so survivorship insurance fits the bill. Because Jane's parents are successful in their own right, Jeff and Susan view this policy as just an extra safety net for Jane, and a way of showing Jane their love and emotional support. Their estate planner and accountant help Jeff and Susan deal with the fact that gifts to the trust won't qualify for the GST gift tax exclusion. Further, they have authorized the trustees of Jane's trust to make distributions to the Society to fund programs and research in the trustee's discretion, after consideration of all other resources available to

Jane. On Jane's death, all remaining insurance proceeds in the trust are to be distributed to the Society. Jeff and Susan understand that there is no tax advantage to these donations, because the funds are outside of their estate, but their goal is to help Jane and the Society, not only to achieve tax benefits.

Charitable Lead Trust

A charitable lead annuity trust (CLAT) was discussed and illustrated earlier within the context of providing benefit to your child with MS and benefit to the Society. For a grandchild, this technique won't be practical because of the GST tax discussed earlier. While many of the technical nuances are beyond the scope of this introduction, and your estate planner and accountant can deal with them, the valuable planning ideas that can help you achieve your personal and charitable goals can still be illustrated. For an eventual gift to a grandchild, your advisors will probably recommend that you use a charitable lead uni-trust (CLUT). A CLUT is a trust designed to benefit charity and, at the same time, provide a future gift (inheritance) to your grandchild at a reduced gift (estate) tax cost. When you set up a CLUT, the Society receives the income (actually a uni-trust payment) for a number of years that you agree to (the longer the number of years, the greater the tax break); thereafter, the assets in the trust are distributed to your grandchild. This is a great mechanism to benefit the Society, protect your grandchild, and achieve tax savings. A uni-trust payment is a fixed percentage of the value of the trust determined each year.

❂ EXAMPLE: You set up a CLUT paying 6.5%. The trust pays the Society 6.5% of the value of the assets each year. If the trust has $1 million in assets, then the Society receives a payment of $65,000. If, next year, the assets grow to $1.2 million the Society receives a payment of 6.5% × $1.2 million, or $78,000.

❂ EXAMPLE: Mary Crane has a substantial estate, is concerned about estate tax, but wants to provide a safety net for her grandson, Bill. She has her estate planner create a 25-year CLUT to which she gifts $1 million. She does not receive a charitable contribution deduction but, for gift tax purposes, her eventual gift to Bill is reduced from $1 million to under $190,000. This reduction results from the payments that will be made to the Society for 25 years. Her accountant will file a gift tax return using up about $190,000 of her gift and GST tax exemptions. The Society will receive an annuity payment each year based on 6.5% of the fair value of the assets in the trust in that year. The first year's payment (assuming a full year) will be $65,000. After the 25th year, the entire value of the trust will be distributed to Bill (or, if Mary prefers, a trust for Bill's benefit). If the trust assets grow at 7.5% year, Bill should receive about $1,150,000. Thus, Mary has provided a significant benefit to the Society and used that benefit to leverage a gift and GST tax beneficial safety net and retirement plan for her grandson.

Using Donations to the Society to Leverage GST Transfers to Benefit Your Grandchildren

Your estate is quite large, and you want to benefit your grandchildren and perhaps later descendants, but the GST tax makes that quite difficult and costly. Unrelated to that objective, you support the Society and its mission to end MS. You can help your grandchildren and benefit the Society simultaneously. To accomplish this, you must combine charitable planning with planning for your grandchildren to avoid the harsh impact of the GST tax. This technique can enable you to provide for the future tuition and medical expenses of your grandchildren without triggering the GST tax that you would cause if you did not combine the charitable gift to the Society with this planning. Since you intended to make charitable donations to the Society in any event, there is no real incremental cost to using this planning to leverage gifts to benefit of your grandchildren.

Assume that you want to pass wealth on to your grandchildren and, in particular, provide for the medical care of a grandchild living with MS. The simple solution would be to set up a trust to pay for your grandchildren's tuition and medical costs and give substantial assets to that trust. However, because the only beneficiaries of such a trust are your grandchildren, every dollar you give to the trust would be subject to the GST tax. In tax parlance, the trust itself would be classified as a "skip person," so that all gifts to it would be subject to GST tax. To avoid this tax cost, you would have to allocate (use up) your GST exemption. Your GST exemption is a tax break that lets you transfer up to a certain amount of assets to grandchildren (or trusts for them) without incurring GST tax. A common theme of planning is to preserve as much of your exemption amounts for later gifts, or at least to save it for situations when it really must be used. If you've already used up your GST exemption, the tax cost of transferring assets to a trust only for your grandchildren would be prohibitive.

So, how can you set up a trust to provide for tuition and medical costs of your grandchildren and not trigger the dreaded GST tax? Because it is assumed that you want to make charitable donations to the Society, you can use this fact to avoid the GST tax on transferring assets to a trust for your grandchildren. How? Structure the trust to benefit the Society as well as your grandchildren. If, for example, you provide that on your death 25% of the trust will be given to the Society, the trust is now designed to benefit a combination of your grandchildren and the organization. The trust will not be classified as a "skip person" for GST tax purposes, thus your gifts to the trust will not trigger the GST tax. Your trustee can be given the discretion to pay medical and tuition expenses for your descendants forever. This can include, for example, all the medical costs of a grandchild with MS. As discussed earlier (see powers of attorney), direct payments of tuition or medical expenses for your grandchildren are not subject to gift or GST tax. In tax terminology, these payments are not treated as taxable distributions from a trust that would trigger GST tax. So, no GST tax is applicable on the gifts you make to the trust by virtue of the inclusion of the Society as a beneficiary (although you'll have to plan with your tax adviser to address all income, GST, and gift tax issues). There is no GST tax on payments of tuition or medical expenses because of the exceptions provided in the tax laws for these payments. On your death, the Society will receive 25% of the trust assets. The trustee will continue to benefit your grandchildren (and even later descendants) by paying trust monies for tuition and medical costs. Tax problem solved. Grandchildren and the Society benefited.

You can take numerous other steps to protect a grandchild with MS and, in many cases, weave in provisions to benefit the Society. These examples illustrate a only few of the many options. The tremendous complexity that the GST tax creates, however, really requires expert advisers and guidance.

Partner/Friend

If you have a friend or partner living with MS that you wish to benefit or protect, or if you have MS and you have a non-married partner, you'll need to address certain legal and tax issues. Planning is quite different for a non-spouse. While some states have domestic partnership laws, most state laws won't provide you the same protection afforded to a spouse. The federal tax laws provide no flexibility or protection for a non-married partner. Some aspects of the planning might be helped by combining the planning with charitable giving but, in all events, you'll need expert local advice. The following discussion reviews possibilities based on some of the estate planning documents you might use in your own planning.

Power of Attorney

This common estate planning document designates a person (agent) to manage your financial, legal, and other affairs if you cannot do so. If you have a non-married partner, it's even more important that you get in place a comprehensive, signed durable power of attorney, because a partner will in most instances not enjoy the same presumptions, or powers under state law, that a spouse would. Thus, the power could be more important to ensure that your partner can assist you if you have an exacerbation. If your partner has MS, you could incorporate specific provisions into your power of attorney permitting your agent to support your partner. Any support or gifts in excess of the annual gift tax exclusion ($12,000 in 2007, but the amount is inflation indexed) will have a gift tax implication. A non-married partner does not qualify for the unlimited gifts that a spouse would. Your agent can also make direct payments for medical or tuition expenses without limit and without gift tax consequences. While you are tailoring your power of attorney to address assisting your partner, give some consideration to having your lawyer modify the gift provisions to include the right to make charitable gifts to the Society.

Revocable Living Trust

Many people use revocable living trusts to avoid probate, although a far more important use is to manage assets during illness or disability. If your family did not support your relationship, using a revocable living trust might enable you and your partner to avoid some of the family entanglements if one of you becomes incapacitated or dies. If you have a revocable living trust as part of your estate plan, be sure to have your attorney make modifications similar to those described for a power of attorney.

Will

Your will should probably include a trust to protect your partner who lives with MS. The trust can provide for the management of assets in the event your partner has reached a point at which she cannot easily manage her own financial affairs. A trust might also ensure some insulation and protection in the event that your family seeks to undermine the bequest. Because bequests to a partner do not qualify for the unlimited estate tax marital deduction, more planning— and more aggressive tax minimization techniques—are necessary. As with all estate planning documents, your will can provide a wonderful opportunity to tailor a charitable bequest. With a non-married partner, a charitable bequest can be a great way to minimize estate tax costs.

> ✪ EXAMPLE: Jane Smith has an estate of $3 million. Her partner, Maureen Jones, has MS. Jane would like to provide protection for Maureen in the event of her death, minimize estate taxes, and benefit the Society. Maureen is insistent on trying to avoid estate tax, not only to minimize taxes, but because of what she views as the unfairness that a non-married partner could face almost a 50% estate tax burden, whereas a married partner has

no estate tax. Jane knows that the first $2 million of her estate will pass to Maureen free of estate tax in 2007 (but that figure may change in the future). Jane wants to minimize the estate tax on the remaining $1 million of her estate while benefiting both Maureen and the Society. To accomplish these goals, Jane provides that, upon her death, $1 million of her estate will be paid to a charitable lead annuity trust (CLAT) to benefit the Society for 20 years, and thereafter to benefit her partner Maureen. If $1 million is given to a 20-year CLAT paying 7.2%, or $72,000, annually to the Society (with payments at the beginning of the year), the value of the eventual gift to Maureen will be reduced to under $100,000. This is because of the 20 years of payments to the Society. The remainder of her estate will, after payments for executor commissions (to Maureen) be paid to Maureen in a lifetime trust. Jane believes the lifetime trust approach will provide Maureen protection if she needs it, but while Maureen is able, she is named as a co-trustee with another friend. The combination of the estate tax exclusion ($2 million in 2007, but may increase or decrease) and the CLAT deduction, will almost eliminate the estate tax. The use of trusts will likely minimize outside interference (e.g., from Jane's family) and protect Maureen. The payments of $72,000 per year to the Society will provide for needed services that Maureen and others can benefit from.

Insurance Trust

The use of insurance trusts is especially common among non-married partners because it provides a safe, non-taxable means of addressing the estate tax (since no marital deduction is available). For non-married partners, especially when one of you has MS, an insurance trust can be used as a means to provide extra protection and address any estate tax issues.

> ✹ EXAMPLE: Michael Jones and Gordon Green are partners. Michael owns a shore home worth several million dollars, as well as other assets. While both Michael and Gordon work full time, Gordon's MS symptoms have progressed, and it is not clear how long he will continue to work. Both Michael and Gordon are concerned about the estate tax that will be due if Michael dies first and leaves the shore home to Gordon. Michael has his estate planner set up an irrevocable life insurance trust, and the trust purchases $2.5 million of insurance on Michael's life. If Michael dies before Gordon, the insurance will fund the payment of the estate tax and ensure enough capital to generate a cash flow to support Gordon in the event he has to stop working. On Gordon's later death, any remaining monies will be given to the Society. If Gordon dies before Michael, Michael will stop paying on the insurance policy, and the trustee will either cash the policy in or sell it in the secondary market, and distribute the proceeds to the Society.

You can take a host of other steps to protect a non-married partner with MS, and often in a manner that supports the Society and the MS community. These examples only illustrated a few of the opportunities.

Chapter Summary

Who do you want to help? Who are you worried about? What is your connection to MS? This chapter has taken the perspective of identifying most of the relationships you might have with someone affected by MS, whether yourself, a spouse, child, grandchild, partner, or other person. You can take affirmative steps to help and protect that person, often in a manner that can benefit the Society. In some situations, your helping the Society can actually enhance the benefits you can provide the person you are seeking to benefit. It can truly be a win-win situation.

> **CAUTION:** Most planning ideas presented in this chapter are complex and must be implemented with the advice of your accountant, estate planning attorney, insurance consultant, investment adviser, wealth manager, and other experts. Be sure to review all the requirements and potential issues and drawbacks to any of the techniques suggested before proceeding.

CHAPTER FOUR

DIFFERENT ASSETS CAN BE USED TO HELP FUND THE CURE

M OST DONORS ASSUME that their choice of how to make a donation is simply of whether to use a check or credit card. While either works, almost any asset can be used to make a donation to the National Multiple Sclerosis Society (the Society). If you consider the wide range of assets that can be donated, and some of the personal, legal, and tax benefits that donating different assets (not just a check) can provide, you might be willing to structure a more sophisticated and larger donation and accomplish several planning objectives.

Sometimes the easiest perspective for you or another prospective donor to take is to focus on a particular asset. You may have a certain asset that you want to sell or give to the Society. You may have read something about a planning technique involving that asset, and you want to explore your options. In many cases, your interest is piqued by a conversation on the golf green about something miraculous your golfing partner achieved by donating a particular asset. This chapter will help you identify some of the planning opportunities available for many of the different assets you are likely to own. We'll start with the most common asset donation: cash.

Cash, Check, Credit Card Payment

The Most Common Donations Are Not Always Simple

A cash donation is the simplest and most common type of gift to the Society. A tax deduction is generally received for the cash contributed. From a practical perspective, cash donations are easy to make. They also are generally simple from a tax perspective—write a check, get a deduction. But alas, in the Alice-in-Wonderland world of tax rules, few things don't have exceptions, special rules, and other twists and turns pertaining to them. Although this book does not focus on tax technicalities, and those covered are confined to Chapter 6, an exception will be made here to illustrate that what you might assume to be a simple cash gift is not always so simple. The take home message is that if some of the other techniques described in this book sound complex, in many cases, they are not that much more complicated than the simple cash donation. This is not to dissuade you from making a donation to the Society by check or credit card, but rather to encourage you not to give up on the more sophisticated planned gifts.

So, you write out a check or give a credit card number to the Society. What issues might affect your deduction?

Donations Reduced by Benefits Received

If a benefit is received in return for the donation, the value of your deduction must be reduced.

> ✪ EXAMPLE: You attend a Society MS Bike Ride and pay $500 to be a sponsor and receive a sponsor jacket. If the fair value of the jacket is $100, you are entitled to a $400 tax deduction.

If you attend a Society gala black tie dinner, for example, the $1,000 you paid for a pair of tickets must be reduced by the cost of the dinner, of which the Society will notify you. There are exceptions for gifts of modest value.

Cash Bequest in Your Will

A cash bequest under your will to the Society is assumed to provide for an estate tax charitable contribution deduction. However, this ignores the reality that very few estates are subject to federal estate tax. The figure is actually less than 1%. So, if you were to make a donation under your will to the Society, unless your estate exceeds $2 million (the estate tax applicable exclusion in 2007, which is scheduled to increase in the future), you will not realize any federal estate tax benefit from the donation. A simple solution might be for you to leave the money you were going to give to the Society to your heirs and ask them to make the donation. They may qualify for an income tax deduction, which is a better tax break than a zero estate tax benefit. If your estate is taxable, a different result may occur.

> ✪ EXAMPLE: For decades, Fran Baker has been a donor to the Society. However, she has never given a significant donation because she wanted to preserve assets for her own needs. She remains worried about the course her MS will take and what types of medical and other care expenses she

may incur that are not covered by insurance. In her will, Fran would like to leave a $100,000 bequest to the Society. When Fran reviews her will with her attorney, her estate is valued at $1.4 million. She lives in a state with no estate tax. The $100,000 will not provide any income or estate tax benefit, but it will increase the legal fees on the administration of her estate. If a bequest is made under Fran's will, the formalities of notifying the charity, obtaining a receipt from the charity, and so on, could easily add $500+ in costs to the administration of her estate. Because Fran's heirs are her three nephews, whom she trusts fully, she opts not to leave the bequest in her will. Instead, she has her attorney add a clause to her power of attorney authorizing her agents to make a donation to the Society in the amount of $100,000. She writes a side letter to her nephews asking them to make sure that the Society receives the $100,000 donation and that, if the full donation wasn't made by her while she was alive and well, or by her agent under her power, they should make donations after her death to the Society in equal one-third amounts, sufficient to bring the total payments up to $100,000. In her letter, she advises them not to count any small donations for annual walk or bike-a-thons as having been paid towards the $100,000 pledge.

Foreign Donations

Donations to foreign charities will generally not qualify for a tax deduction. If you want to fund a foreign MS research project, you may be able to accomplish your charitable and tax goals by making a gift to the Society and requesting that they fund the overseas project. If the Society is willing and able to make the commitment, your donation will be fully deductible, and you will achieve your charitable goals. Many foreign charities have U.S. qualified charities that raise money for them (called feeder organizations). This may be another option,

When Is Your Donation Deductible?

If you write a check out to the Society, it's deductible in the year you mail it or unconditionally give it to the organization, so long as it clears the bank in due course. If you make a payment by credit card, your donation is deductible in the year you incur the charge, even if you pay the actual credit card bill in a later year. So, if you're looking to get a deduction in late December, you might be better off using a credit card, or if you send a check, using certified mail to prove the mailing date.

Numerous other restrictions and limitations affect cash and all other donations. An overview of some of these technicalities is presented in Chapter 6.

Deferred or Planned Cash Donations

Cash donations can also be planned and paid over time, so that you can make a more significant current commitment without undue financial pressure.

> ✪ EXAMPLE: Judy Frank is tremendously appreciative of all the help that her local Society chapter has provided for her since her recent diagnosis. She wants to send a big thank-you to the volunteers and professionals at the chapter, but her financial resources are somewhat limited. She signs a pledge agreement for a $10,000 pledge, payable at the rate of $1,000/year, but which she anticipates paying at the rate of $2,500/year over four years. This enables her to send that big "thank you" and make a contribution that really makes her feel good.

Life Insurance

Great Way to Make a Larger Contribution

You would really like to make a long-term and meaningful commitment to the Society, but don't have the financial strength to write a big check today. Don't give up the thought of a larger donation: You may be able use life insurance to accomplish your goal in an affordable manner. It's a great "feel good" way to help the Society. Insurance can provide a great example of giving back for your children and others who look to you for guidance.

Buy a New Policy for the Society

You can buy a permanent insurance policy that the Society owns and for which the Society is named beneficiary. Each year, you make a contribution to the Society sufficient to pay the premium. You get an income tax charitable contribution deduction for the gift. The Society owns the policy, pays the premium, and eventually is the beneficiary. In the meantime, the cash value of the policy grows as an asset. You'll have made a large gift that you can pay over time. But don't reduce your annual gifts to the Society because of this: The insurance policy should be an additional gift, because the Society won't be getting current dollars that it can use from the premium payments.

> ✪ EXAMPLE: John Smith's sister Julie has MS. John doesn't have the financial wherewithal to make a large gift to the Society, but wants to show his sister support. John, age 30, applies for a $100,000 life insurance policy, naming the Society as owner and beneficiary. The premiums for a policy that

will be fully paid in 10 years are only $1,002 per year. Each year, John donates $1,002 to the Society, which pays the premium. After a 40% income tax deduction, John's out-of-pocket cost for a $100,000 bequest in honor of his sister Julie is only about $600/year.

Donate an Existing Policy

Instead of having a new policy purchased by you in the name of the Society, you could donate to the organization an existing policy that you no longer need.

⊕ EXAMPLE: Jason Cutter's youngest child just graduated college. Jason has several insurance policies, including an old $500,000 universal life policy, which he had purchased to ensure adequate resources for his children's college costs. Since his family's need for the policy has been obviated, Jason donates the policy to the Society. While Jason might be able to sell the policy to investors, he's uncomfortable with unknown investors owning an insurance policy on his life and therefore prefers the charitable route.

Restrictions and Issues Affect Insurance Donations

Many considerations can affect your insurance planning, some of which are noted here. These issues highlight a common cautionary thread throughout this book: You need professional guidance to implement any planning ideas. You cannot have any rights (incidence of ownership) in the insurance policy you donate. If you do, your contributions to pay for the policy will not qualify as tax deductions. Before completing the donation of any insurance policy, have your estate planner confirm that the Society can legally own (have an insurable interest in) an insurance policy on your life under state law. When donating an insurance policy, your income tax charitable contribution deduction will probably be based on the premiums you previously paid into the policy. You may not qualify for a contribution deduction for the full fair market value of the policy. Be wary of more complex charitable insurance plans, because many of them are fraught with problems. Some problematic plans include arrangements whereby a charity partners with an investor group to buy insurance on your life to profit both the investors and the charity. There are many variations on this scheme, and caution must be exercised. Clearing any charitable insurance plan with your attorney and the Society before proceeding will assure both you and the Society that the plan will succeed without creating tax and legal problems you're not looking for.

Marketable Securities
Donating Appreciated Securities

You can always sell stocks and donate the proceeds to the Society. It's simple, but not always the best tax result. When you donate stock, your contribution deduction is based on the fair value of the stock donated. Publicly traded stock is valued at the average of the highest and lowest selling price on the date you make the contribution.

> ✪ EXAMPLE: Fran West has owned stock in a well known bank for years. The stock was purchased at $20 per share and is now worth $140 per share. Fran could sell the stock and donate the proceeds to the Society, but she would pay a capital gains tax on the gain of $120 share. Instead, Fran directs her broker to transfer the stock to the Society: a simple no-cost process. Fran has no capital gains to report because she sold no stock. Fran, however, can claim a charitable contribution deduction on her personal income tax return of $140 per share.

Don't Donate Depreciated Securities

The tax benefits and simplicity of donating appreciated stock make it an ideal way to benefit the Society and yourself. However, don't assume that all stock donations are beneficial. If you own stock that has declined in value and donate it, you won't benefit from any of the loss for tax purposes. For losers, you're better off selling the security, recognizing your capital loss for income tax purposes (for whatever benefit you can get), and donating as much of the cash proceeds as you wish to the Society.

For Really Big Gains, Consider a Charitable Remainder Trust

If you have really substantial gains on a large stock position, more sophisticated planning is called for.

⚙ EXAMPLE: Steve North purchased 100,000 shares of a start-up research company, Myelin Repair, Inc. (MRI), for $1 per share. The company has developed a new drug that has just received FDA approval, and the stock price has shot up to $57 per share on an unadjusted basis. Steve's gain is huge, $5.6 million. The stock pays almost no dividends. Steve is retiring and needs more income to cover living expenses. He also wishes to diversify this investment holding, because it has become such a substantial portion of his estate. However, to sell his MRI stock would trigger substantial capital gains. Steve works out a more comprehensive plan. Steve will contribute 40,000 shares, worth $2,240,000, to an exchange fund sponsored by a major investment firm. This will enable him to receive income tax–free limited partnership interests, diversify his portfolio, and have an asset that is ideally suited for other family estate tax planning transactions. Steve will sell 20,000 shares at $1,120,000 and pay capital gains tax. This will provide him with a cash pool to use as he wishes. Steve will retain 20,000 shares because he still likes MRI's prospects. Steve will donate 20,000 shares to a charitable remainder trust (CRT), which he will structure to provide a 5% payout. The CRT shares will be sold income tax–free by the trust, and the proceeds reinvested by the trust in a diversified portfolio. Steve will receive back a quarterly payment of $14,000 for the rest of his life. Steve will realize a charitable contribution deduction of $555,236, which will help offset the gain on the sale of his MRI shares. Most importantly, Steve will be sharing some of his windfall with the Society and helping them fund a research project with MRI as part of the organization's program to partner with members of the investment community to fuel MS research. Because of his charitable goals, Steve structured the CRT with only a 5% payout to himself. He anticipates that his wealth manager will earn at least 6.5% on the CRT investments. Thus, at the end of Steve's life expectancy, the Society should receive in excess of $1.7 million. The financial and charitable benefits are significant.

Personal Property

The ability to donate personal property, such as art, jewelry, furniture, cars, and so forth, opens up new opportunities for donations to help the Society in its mission to end MS. Here, we'll review some of the planning opportunities and rules for these types of donations.

Donating Tangible Property

Gifts of personal property are simple to describe, and they may be simple to conclude, but personal-property gifts are subject to a myriad of restrictions and reporting requirements. Personal property includes items such as furniture, artwork, jewelry, and so forth (not land or buildings). Detailed rules are provided for the appraisal of property contributions, reporting requirements (which vary based on the nature and value of the property donated), restrictions on deductions for personal property (limited to a percentage of your income, etc.), and more (see Chapter 6). Although you can deduct the current value (fair market value) of many of the assets you contribute to the Society, this is not always the case with tangible personal property. These rules should not deter you from donating tangible property: Rather, they should simply encourage you to keep your accountant involved in monitoring the process and its consequences.

Clothing and Household Items

Contributions of clothing and household items must be in good used condition or better. Items of modest value may, by regulation, be denied any deduction. Paintings, antiques, art, jewelry, and items valued over $500, for which a qualified appraisal is obtained, are excluded from these new restrictions. A detailed list and photographs of any such items should be retained.

Donating Tangible Property Unrelated to the Society's Tax-Exempt Purpose

Property Whose Use Is Not Related to the Society's Tax-Exempt Function: If you contribute appreciated tangible property, such as a painting, to the Society, your income tax deduction will be limited to what you paid for the property (your adjusted tax basis), not the fair market value of the property, if the property's use by the Society is not related to its tax-exempt purpose or function.

Property Whose Use Is Related to the Society's Tax-Exempt Function: If you contribute appreciated tangible property, and the property's use by the Society is related to its tax-exempt purpose or function, such as furniture used in an MS center waiting room, your income tax deduction will be the fair market value of the property (not just what you paid for it). However, if the Society disposes of the property within three years of your contribution, your income tax charitable contribution benefit will be adjusted downward from fair value back to your cost (adjusted basis), unless the Society certifies that the property was to be used for furthering its purpose or function, but that use became impossible to implement.

Fractional Interests in Personal Property

Although you can donate a fractional interest in tangible personal property, such as a painting, the restrictions on these donations are so severe that it is not likely to be a practical approach. If you donated a fractional interest in personal property to the Society, the organization must receive full ownership prior to the earlier of your death (get out the Ouija board) or 10 years. If you make a later contribution of the balance of the property to the Society, your deduction for income, gift, and estate tax purposes is the lesser of value at the time of your initial contribution or the value at the date of your subsequent contribution. If the value of the property increases, your deduction remains limited to the earlier value.

Retirement Plan Assets

Bequests of IRA and Retirement Plan Assets

IRA and other retirement plan assets are great assets to use to fund a bequest to the Society. On your death, if your estate is large enough, retirement plan assets are subject to a double tax: income tax on eventual distribution to your heirs and estate tax. Although with careful planning the income tax costs can be stretched out and the tax deferred, and to some extent estate taxes mitigated by using IRA and retirement plan assets to fund estate tax–oriented trusts, the benefit of donating these assets remains substantial. This is a great way to benefit the Society with an asset that might net only a very small percentage of dollars to your heir after all taxes are considered. Also, it avoids any issues of your needing the money during your lifetime, so it's a great charitable giving technique if you are living with the challenges of MS. If your spouse lives with MS, the same technique can be used, but the Society would be the remainder beneficiary after your spouse dies.

The method in which to make such a donation is to name the Society as a beneficiary of the IRA or other retirement plan that you wish to donate. This planning can be facilitated by the following:

- Consider splitting your IRA account so that you have the Society as the sole beneficiary of one account. For example, if you have a $1 million IRA, and want to leave $500,000 to your only daughter and $500,000 to the Society, split the IRA and name the Society as beneficiary of one account and your daughter as the beneficiary of the other.
- Sign a beneficiary designation listing the "National Multiple Sclerosis Society" as beneficiary.
- Have your advisers determine whether your spouse must provide a written consent to your leaving your retirement plan to the Society instead of him or her.

- Sign a pledge form with the Society so that they are alerted to your intent and commitment.
- Revise your power of attorney to clearly exclude from your agent the power to change the beneficiary designation for the IRA or retirement plan involved.
- Review the planning with your financial planner and accountant. You might opt to purchase life insurance to supplement the inheritance to your heirs, or take other steps. Also, they can review the many technical nuances of this type of planning with you.
- Be certain that the use of IRA or retirement plan assets is carefully planned. For example, if your executor (personal representative) satisfies a specific dollar charitable bequest under your will (pecuniary bequest) with an IRA, taxable income could inadvertently be triggered and your hoped for tax benefits defeated. This is because, if your executor satisfied a pecuniary bequest with retirement assets subject to income tax (income in respect of a decedent, or IRD), gain must be recognized. Instead, make the Society a specific beneficiary of your IRA, or have a provision in your will or trust mandating the use of your IRA to pay your bequest to the Society.

Lifetime Donation of IRA and Retirement Plan Assets

The flexibility of permitting donors to contribute IRA funds to charities while the donors are alive is a long-sought benefit by many charities. Congress finally provided some relief, but the window for this benefit was only enacted for 2006–2007, although there is hope that the benefit will be extended to future years or made permanent. This benefit has a host of technical requirements, including the need for the plan sponsor's cooperation.

- This leniency provision only applies to IRAs, not other types of plans.
- Individuals age 70.5 or older may gift up to $100,000 in each of 2006 and 2007 to the Society. You must have passed your half birthday before consummating the donation. It is not sufficient that the donation be made in the year that you turn 70.5.
- The donation must be made directly from the plan trustee to the Society to qualify.
- The donation must have otherwise qualified to be deductible-in-full as a charitable contribution deduction.
- You must obtain a written confirmation of the donation and that no goods or services were received in exchange for it.
- Except for this new rule, the distribution from the IRA would have to be included in your gross income to qualify. If you meet all the requirements, the IRA donation is not included in your income. The result is that any limitations on contributions won't limit the tax benefit of such a contribution. This issue had been a significant deterrent to charitable gifts of IRA assets in that the entire IRA distribution may have been taxable, but only a portion deductible, thus generating an income tax cost for trying to make a contribution. The limitations on charitable contributions based on your adjusted gross income (AGI) discussed in Chapter 6

are a prime factor in this. Another problem was the phase-out of itemized deductions based on gross income. The inclusion in gross income of IRA funds withdrawn could thus result in a decrease in other deductions.

- The donations will count toward any required minimum distributions.
- The amount of IRA qualified charitable distribution does not also provide a contribution deduction. The charity cannot be a donor-advised fund, supporting organization, or split-interest entity. Thus, only public charities, such as the Society, qualify for this benefit.

Although the benefits of this provision are tremendous, the restrictions and limitations make its use very limited. Hopefully, Congress will see fit to expand this benefit, make the requirements more reasonable, and make it a permanent fixture of the tax laws.

Family and Closely Held Businesses

Family and closely held (a few owners) equity (stock in a corporation, membership interests in a limited liability company, etc.) can present many unique and valuable charitable giving opportunities.

Business Inventory

Inventory can be a great donation to support the Society and the MS community. Donating bottled water, hats, or other items to a local chapter's walk or bike event can be a tremendous help in building the excitement and success of the event. What type of deduction can you obtain for donating inventory? The general rule is that when the property, if sold, would generate ordinary income (not capital gains), your charitable contribution deduction is limited. The limitation is the lesser of the fair value of the property you donate, or what you paid for the property (adjusted tax basis). Because the amount of your deduction is limited to what you paid for the property, the complex rules about whether the Society used the property for its exempt purpose (which apply to donations of tangible property such as art) are not relevant. If your corporation donates inventory to the Society in the year it is manufactured, your corporation claims its deduction as part of its cost of goods sold, not as a charitable contribution deduction. This is a valuable benefit in that corporate contributions are limited to 10% of income, but deductions as cost of goods sold are not limited at all. If you're a sole proprietor, this deduction as a cost of goods sold can save you self-employment taxes.

A special rule permits a larger deduction if the inventory is donated for the care of the ill, need of minors, or if the inventory is used in the Society's exempt purpose. Qualifying donations permit you to deduct your cost (tax basis), plus half of the appreciation (but not more than twice your cost).

Charitable Bail Out of Closely Held Stock

Donations to the Society, or a charitable remainder trust to benefit the Society, can have special use when a key asset is stock in a closely held business. A charitable bail-out of a closely held business' stock can address important planning problems for a closely held business owner. Stock in a closely held corporation can be difficult or impossible to sell, because outsiders will generally be very reluctant to own a minority interest in a close corporation. Another problem could relate to the type of corporation involved. Assume that the corporation is a C corporation (i.e., not an S corporation) and has available cash that you would like to donate to the Society. However, it may not be practical to make a dividend distribution to provide the cash for such a donation, because a dividend distribution will result in double taxation (the corporation first pays tax on the earnings and then you pay tax again on the receipt of the net earnings in the form of a dividend). Another common problem scenario for a closely held business is when a parent owns stock in a close corporation and wishes to transfer control to a child without triggering income tax on redemption. One possible solution for this latter scenario is called a stock bail-out. You can make a gift of any portion of the stock in your corporation to a charity. At some later date, the charity may, of its sole discretion, sell some of this stock back to your corporation. This provides you with a charitable contribution deduction for income tax purposes for the stock donated. The Society can eventually receive a cash amount for the contribution. When the corporation redeems the stock, the interest of the children owning stock will increase, because the charitable bail-out/redemption of your stock will increase their relative ownership interest.

⊗ EXAMPLE: Paul Woods owns stock in a family manufacturing business. Over the years, he has made gifts of stock, using the annual gift tax exclusion, to his three children who are actively involved in the business. Paul now owns about 60% of the stock, and he would like to reduce his ownership below 50%. Paul has the corporation appraised, as well as the value of a 12% interest in the corporation. Paul could sell the stock to his children, but that would trigger capital gains tax and would add assets (i,e., the cash received from a sale) back to his estate, which is inconsistent with his estate planning objectives. Paul confers with the Society. After appropriate due diligence, representations, and warranties from Paul, and an opinion from tax counsel, the Society agrees to accept the donation. Paul then makes a donation of 12% of the outstanding stock to the Society. At some later date, the Society may choose to sell some of this stock back to the corporation. These steps could provide Paul with a charitable contribution deduction for the stock donated. When Paul's corporation repurchases stock from the Society, that stock becomes treasury stock, and it is no longer relevant to the determination of ownership percentages in the company. This reduces Paul's ownership to

54.5% [60% – 12%/100% – 12%], close to his goal. A few more annual gifts of stock might suffice to complete the reduction of his ownership interests to less than 50%. The Society should eventually be able to receive cash if it sells the stock back to the Corporation.

A number of issues must be addressed with this type of planning. The Society cannot be obligated to sell any portion of the stock back to the corporation. All sales must be at its discretion. If a pre-arranged plan for the resale of the stock exists, it can be difficult to differentiate whether the Society was so obligated. If the Society is not under any legal obligation to resell the stock it receives, there is a possibility that it could sell the stock to another person (even one of your competitors), vote the shares in a manner inconsistent with your desires, and so on. This technique can also be use for S corporations. Properly planned, a charitable bail-out can be a helpful technique.

Business Advertising Expense

A commonly overlooked opportunity might simplify and enhance your deductions for supporting the Society. In some instances, you might be able to characterize cash payments or property donations to the Society as business advertising expenses. This might prove valuable, because it avoids the numerous and complex rules and limitations that affect charitable contribution deductions. If the payments your business makes to the Society bear a direct relationship to your business, and these payments were made with the reasonable expectation of a financial return commensurate with the payments, the amounts can be deducted as business advertising (an ordinary and necessary trade or business expense).

Principal Residence or Farm

Generally, you can only obtain a charitable contribution deduction if you donate your entire interest in a particular property to the Society. There are several exceptions, including an important one relating to your home. You can make a donation today of an interest in your personal residence or farm that only takes effect in the future. This special rule permits you to claim a current income tax deduction, without the legal costs and complications of setting up a trust to do so. Thus, you can contribute your house to the Society and continue to live in it for the remainder of your life, or for some set number of years that you choose. Your spouse could also reside in the residence as well. The gift of the house to the Society, however, must be permanent (irrevocable). You can use these rules to donate your house, cooperative apartment, or even vacation home to the Society. A donation of a remainder interest in a farm, which includes land and buildings, also qualifies. Donations of fixtures, furniture, and other personal assets in the house or on the farm will not qualify.

✪ EXAMPLE: Donna Ford has MS. She resides in a ranch house that is completely accessible. She hopes to continue to live in her home for the rest of her life. Because she is single and has no children to whom she wants to leave her house, her hope is to help the Society finance research on improved MRI technology to better ascertain axonal damage, not just damage to myelin. As her MS has progressed, and her savings have grown, she realizes that it's an opportune time to sell her retail business. She feels it is becoming too hard to work the hours necessary, and that the value of the business has grown to the point that it should fund her early retirement. Donna donates her home to the Society, retaining a life estate, which gives her the right to live in her home for the remainder of her life. The income tax deduction she realizes on the donation of the remainder interest in her home offsets some of the tax cost she will incur on selling her business. Thus, Donna is able to bank more of the proceeds from the sale of her business for her retirement, while assuring a wonderful future gift for the Society.

The value of your income tax deduction for donating a remainder interest in your home or farm is rather complex to calculate, and you'll want the assistance of your accountant. The deduction will consider that portion of the donation classified as land value, and that portion classified as building value.

Commercial Real Estate

Real estate is a common asset used in more complex charitable plans. A host of special issues and provisions affect real estate donations. The following discussion summarizes a few of them. An important threshold issue is that, in light of all the problems that can arise with property subject to hazardous waste or other litigation issues, the Society, as would any charity, will not accept a donation of real estate until it has had ample time to perform due diligence and make sure that no title, environmental, or other problems exist. State transfer and deed taxes may not apply to transfers of real estate to a charitable organization. This can provide a substantial savings when compared to an actual sale. If you own real properties in several states directly (rather than through a limited liability company, partnership, or other entity), your estate will face ancillary probate in those other states and, depending on that state's tax system, additional estate or inheritance tax. If a property is instead donated to the Society, even in the form of a charitable remainder trust so that you will receive a continued income (cash flow) stream, the ancillary probate and tax problem is avoided.

If the property being donated was depreciated (writing off a portion of the purchase price each year over the time period permitted by the tax laws), then depreciation recapture (recharacterization of some portion of the gain attributable to depreciation) can cause additional problems by reducing the amount of your charitable contribution deduction. This technicality should be reviewed with your accountant.

If you donate real estate to your private foundation, rather than to the Society (which is a public charity), you might not qualify for a deduction equal to the full value of the property donated. Donations to the Society are not subject to this limitation. Your income tax deduction is limited in the case of certain capital gain property.

Real estate contributions in which the property has appreciated are subject to a limitation that your deduction cannot exceed 30% of your adjusted gross income. An exception exists: If you donate real estate to a public charity, like the Society, a special election can be made to reduce your contribution deduction by the amount of gain that would have been classified as long-term capital gain (see Chapter 6). If the property is donated to a private charity, a 20% limitation applies.

A donation of real estate subject to a mortgage is treated as a part gift/part sale. The amount of mortgage on the property that the donor is relieved of is treated as an amount realized as if the property were sold. This rule applies even when non-recourse financing is used.

✪ EXAMPLE: Steven Cane owns a small retail strip shopping center worth $1 million, which he developed at a cost of $765,000. His adjusted tax basis in the property (cost to build less depreciation) is only $100,000. Steven donates the property to the Society, subject to a non-recourse first mortgage of $500,000. Steven is treated as if he sold the property and realized $500,000, the amount of the mortgage, less an allocable share of his $100,000 basis. The basis is allocated using the relative values of the mortgage and the fair market value of the property. Because the mortgage of $500,000 is one-half the value of the $1 million value, 50% of the developer's adjusted basis of $100,00 ($50,000) is allocated against the amount realized. Thus, Steven has a gain of $450,000 [$500,000 − ($500,000/$1,000,000 × $100,000)] on making the donation.

✪ EXAMPLE: Lissette Norman purchased investment land many years ago for $200,000, taking out a $150,000 mortgage to complete the purchase. The mortgage has been paid down to $100,000. The property is now worth $1 million, and Lissette wants to donate it to the Society to use for a new research facility that will be conducting research financed by private-equity partnership. Lissette is deemed to have received proceeds on the donation of $100,000, the amount of the mortgage. These proceeds are offset by a pro-rata portion of Lissette's $200,000 tax basis of $20,000 [$100,000 mortgage/$1,000,000 fair value × $200,000 basis].

Generally, a donor cannot obtain a deduction for a charitable contribution of less than an entire interest in property.

✪ EXAMPLE: Dana Smith permits a local Society chapter to use his vacant land for overflow parking. The value of this use can readily be estimated from prices of nearby parking facilities. No deduction is permitted, since this is a donation of a non-qualifying partial interest in property.

This exception does not apply where the partial interest is the entire interest of the donor. An undivided part interest in property can qualify for a charitable contribution deduction. For example, a donation of 10 acres of a 35-acre parcel, or 40% of an income interest in a property in which you don't have any other interests will qualify without this limit. Special rules apply to remainder interests in a personal residence or farm (see the earlier discussion).

Chapter Summary

Whatever real estate, business, or other assets you own and are willing to use to benefit the Society, a charitable plan can be created to achieve optimal tax savings for you and your loved ones, meet other personal goals you might have, and benefit the Society and its important goals. Each asset creates its own charitable giving issues and opportunities. This chapter has surveyed many common assets and hopefully given you ideas on how you can use different assets to benefit the Society.

CHAPTER FIVE

MEET PERSONAL GOALS WHILE FUNDING THE CURE

WHAT GOALS AND OBJECTIVES motivate your charitable, financial, and estate planning? Benefiting charity can be a presumed goal of any compassionate or caring person. However, if your other goals and objectives can be met while simultaneously benefiting the National Multiple Sclerosis Society (the Society), your willingness and ability to contribute should be even greater. If you can identify the specific goals you have, the concerns that worry you, and the objectives you want to meet, a plan can often be crafted to accomplish several of your goals. With some creativity, even goals that appear, on the surface, to be inconsistent can be melded into a single plan that substantially meets all of them. Chapter 3 evaluated ways to coordinate charitable giving to benefit specific people who are important to you. Chapter 4 evaluated ways to use specific assets to accomplish personal and charitable goals. This chapter evaluates the common goals many major donors to the Society have had, perhaps providing you with some ideas and guidance about how you can meet similar goals.

Ensuring You'll Have Enough Cash Flow (Income)

For many prospective donors, the key impediment to making a larger gift—and a key planning goal when structuring a large donation—is to ensure the donor adequate cash flow for personal needs. If this is a concern for you, in many cases, using a charitable remainder trust (CRT) or a gift annuity may suffice to accomplish your dual goals of preserving your cash flow while supporting the Society.

Using a Charitable Remainder Trust to Create Cash Flow

A CRT can be a tremendous estate and financial planning vehicle to generate cash flow. A CRT is a charitable trust to which you contribute assets, typically appreciated assets. You obtain a current income charitable contribution deduction based on the expected value of the eventual donation to the Society, which generates cash flow. The CRT can sell the appreciated assets you donate without triggering any tax. That preserves cash flow. Finally, the CRT can pay you a periodic payment for a specified number of years or for your life. That provides cash flow that could be used to meet your living expenses. An example illustrates this plan:

> ❂ EXAMPLE: Mike Fitzgerald, whose brother has MS, purchased XYZ, Inc. stock in 2001 for $10 per share. The value per share is now $1,000. The stock pays almost no dividends. Mike is retiring, and needs more income to cover living expenses. He also wishes to diversify his XYZ, Inc. holdings because they have become such a substantial portion of his estate. However, to sell XYZ, Inc. stock would trigger a substantial capital gains tax. Mike also is interested in helping fund additional services for those with MS. Mike could instead donate the stock to a CRT and receive back a monthly payment for life (and even for the life of his wife as well). The Society could sell the stock and invest in a diversified portfolio designed to generate cash flow. The Society

should not have to recognize any capital gains tax of $990/share on the sale. As a result, Mike can effectively have the entire investment, undiminished by capital gains tax, working to generate his monthly income. If Mike and his wife are age 65, a CRT could pay them $65,000/year in installments for life. They would also receive a charitable deduction of $213,665. The financial benefits are potentially tremendous. While Mike could also consider other techniques like an exchange fund, those approaches may not accomplish his charitable goals.

Gift Annuities Generate Cash Flow

Gift annuities are a popular form of charitable giving and, in many respects, are simplified versions of the CRT just discussed. You could make a donation of appreciated stock (and avoid the capital gains tax) or a gift of cash to the Society in exchange for a payment of a fixed amount (an annuity) for your life. You can even structure the gift annuity to pay a regular amount to you and your spouse for your joint lives. Unlike a CRT, you can arrange for a gift annuity directly with the Society, without the complexity or legal costs associated with a CRT.

If you donate appreciated property to the Society in exchange for a gift annuity, you will recognize a portion of the taxable gain that you would have realized had the property been sold, over time as you receive annuity payments. You'll also obtain a current charitable contribution deduction dependent on your age, life expectancy, and other factors (actuarial calculations).

How to Donate Property Worth More Than You Can Afford to Give Away

In some instances, you may not wish to donate the entire asset involved and instead want some payment or value in return. This could simply be based on your need for some portion of the asset you want to donate to meet your retirement or other financial goals. No problem. You can donate any portion of the asset you wish, and this control and flexibility can be a great tool for you to convert an asset that doesn't produce cash flow into a contribution deduction and some cash. These goals can be achieved with a bargain sale to the Society.

> ❂ EXAMPLE: Nancy Payne owns a parcel of land worth $1 million, and she sells it to the Society for $200,000. The results are easiest to understand if the donor, Nancy views it as two independent transactions: A charitable gift and a sale. Nancy should qualify for a charitable contribution deduction for the gift portion of the real property donation, $800,000. She should report a sale (perhaps a capital gain on the excess of the proceeds over her allocable basis) for the sale portion of $200,000.

✿ EXAMPLE: James Pearson, a real estate developer, donates land worth $1.4 million to the Society, but wishes to receive some money in return. James' investment (adjusted tax basis) in the property is only $200,000. James sells one-half of the property to the Society for $700,000 (one-half of an undivided interest), and he donates the remaining one-half interest to the Society. The results of a part sale, part gift are as follows (assuming James resides in a state with no income tax): The proceeds from the bargain sale of half of the property to the Society is $700,000. The income tax cost to the donor, assuming a 35% federal tax rate and no state income taxes, is estimated at $210,000 [35% of ($700,000 − 1/2 x 200,000)]. The net of tax proceeds are thus $490,000 ($700,000 − $210,000). In addition, James realizes an income tax benefit from that half of the property donated to the Society of $245,000 ($700,000 × 35%). How does this compare to a sale and later donation by James to the organization? The consequences—if the donor instead sold the property for $1.4 million, retained the $700,000 desired, and donated the balance to the Society—would be less favorable. The proceeds of $1,400,000 would be reduced by the costs of the sale (commissions, fees local tax, and transfer taxes), estimated at $180,000. Net proceeds would be $1,220,000. Federal, State, and local income taxes (assuming an effective combined rate of 35%) would be $427,000. The net proceeds after costs and taxes would be $793,000. If James then retained the desired funds of $700,000, the balance available for contribution would only be $93,000. James would realize a contribution deduction for this amount.

Creating a Retirement Plan Using Charitable Giving

Charitable giving can be used in several ways to create the equivalent of a retirement plan. A special type of charitable remainder trust, called a net income make-up uni-trust (NIM-CRUT) can be used to benefit the Society and create the equivalent of a retirement plan for yourself. A charitable lead trust (CLT) can be used to create something analogous to a retirement plan for your child.

Charitable Remainder Uni-trust As a Retirement Plan

A CRT was described in previous chapters. In simple terms, a typical CRT arrangement has you contribute appreciated stock to the CRT. The CRT sells the stock and does not pay capital gains tax, because a CRT is tax exempt. The CRT then invests the proceeds and pays you an annuity for life. A couple of spins on this "plain vanilla" CRT can turn a CRT into a means of providing a retirement plan–like benefit to you, all while still benefiting the Society. First, some background.

A CRT can be structured as an annuity trust (CRAT) that pays you a fixed amount each year of your life. If you gave $1 million to a CRAT structured to pay a 6% annuity, you would receive $60,000 every year. A CRT can also be structured as a uni-trust (a charitable remainder uni-trust or CRUT) that pays an amount each year based on a fixed percentage of each year's value of the CRUT's assets. So, if the 6% CRUT paid the same $60,000 in its first year, if the stocks it held increased to $1,500,000 by next year, the CRUT would pay you 6% of this figure, or $90,000. A couple of additional twists to go.

A CRUT can also be structured as an income-only uni-trust. This modified form of CRUT can be used to provide you an "income-only arrangement." Using this type of CRUT, you, as the income beneficiary, only receive the actual trust income if the income is less than the fixed percentage payment required (e.g., 6% of the principal of the trust). This type of trust can also include a "make-up provision." This is called a net income make-up CRUT, or NIM-CRUT. In early years, actual income might be less than the 6% required CRUT payment. In later years, if the net income of the CRUT exceeds the specified percentage of trust assets required to be paid (e.g., 6%), this excess can then be paid to you—as the income beneficiary—to make up for the shortfall in prior years. The shortfall is determined based on the difference between the amounts actually paid in prior years, and the amounts that were required to have been paid based on the fixed percentage. The key is to intentionally fund a CRUT with assets that won't generate much income initially, coupled with this make-up of the shortfall after your retirement. This concept can best be illustrated with an example.

✪ EXAMPLE: Daniel Williams has a substantial income, is getting on in years, and wishes to provide for his favorite charity, the National Multiple Sclerosis Society (the Society). Daniel expects to retire in five years. Upon retirement, Daniel expects his income to drop significantly, placing him in a lower income tax bracket. Daniel establishes a net-income-only charitable remainder uni-trust arrangement with a make-up provision (a NIM-CRUT). Daniel funds the trust with a $1 million initial contribution. Daniel receives a current income tax deduction while he is in his prime earning years and highest marginal tax bracket. The trustee of the CRUT invests the $1 million in low-dividend–paying growth stocks. The uni-trust percentage is set at the lowest permissible amount that complies with tax law requirements, or 5%. The dividends on the stock portfolio produce a mere 0.75% return, or $7,500, which is paid to Daniel. After year five, Daniel retires. The stock portfolio, which has appreciated to $1.5 million, is liquidated and invested in high-yield bond instruments, REITs, and other income-oriented investments. These income investments produce a cash return of 8%, or $120,000. Daniel is entitled to distributions of 5% of the $1.5 million CRUT asset value based on the uni-trust amount provided, or $75,000. However, as a result of the make-up provision, Daniel can be paid additional amounts in each of the remaining years of the trust to make-up for the shortfall in prior, pre-retirement years.

Daniel's shortfall would have totaled $212,500. This is the excess of what Daniel should have been paid had the CRUT produced enough income: [(5 years × (5% × $1 million value)] = $50,000 (ignoring growth), over what Daniel actually received in each of those years (5 years × $7,500). Daniel will be entitled to all the income from the income-only uni-trust for a number of years to come, until this shortfall is repaid. Once it is repaid, Daniel will still be entitled to 5% of the value of the CRUT in each year. By having deferred $212,500 of income to his retirement years, Daniel may save income taxes because of his lower post-retirement income tax bracket. He has also shifted significant income to a time period when he will need it.

A Charitable Lead Trust Can Create a Retirement Plan for Your Child

A charitable lead trust (CLT) is a technique generally used to minimize the gift tax costs on large transfers to your children. In some instances, a CLT can be structured to be taxed to you (a grantor trust) so that you can realize a contribution deduction for the donations it makes. However, a CLT can also be used in a manner intended to generate something akin to a retirement plan for your child.

✪ EXAMPLE: Marsha Smith has a daughter with MS, age 25, who is presently working. Marsha is concerned that, because of fatigue and other symptoms, her daughter is unlikely to be able to work to a typical retirement age of 65. Marsha is also keenly aware of recent advances in medical research that show promise of helping her daughter. Marsha establishes a CLT to pay a fixed 7% amount, $70,000, annually to the Society each year for the next 25 years. The payments over this term of years eliminate almost any gift tax impact on Marsha's transferring $1 million to the CLT (the present value of the gift is reduced to about $70,000). In 25 years, when her daughter is age 50, the CLT ends, and an early retirement plan will be available to help her. Marsha anticipates that the $1 million should increase substantially before her daughter's anticipated retirement at age 50. Meanwhile, Marsha is optimistic that the $70,000/year to the Society will help fund valuable research efforts.

Create a Safety Net for Family Medical Expenses

You can set up a trust to provide a safety net to cover medical costs of your entire family, while avoiding the costly generation-skipping transfer (GST) tax and still benefiting the Society. This concept was discussed in Chapter 2 and is illustrated here with an example.

✪ EXAMPLE: Mark Johnson has his estate planner structure a trust to benefit his grandchildren and later descendants, and the Society. On Mark's death, 25% of the trust assets (the corpus) will be given to the Society as a donation. Prior to Mark's death, all the trust will be available to pay for medical expenses for his descendants. After Mark's death, the three-quarters of the trust assets remaining after the donation to the Society will continue to be used forever to pay for medical costs for his grandchildren and later descendants. This trust will be formed in a state that has eliminated any laws limiting the duration for which a trust can last (rule against perpetuities). The trustee Mark names will be given the discretion to pay medical expenses for his grandchildren and future descendants at his discretion. This can include, for example, all the medical costs of a grandchild with MS. These direct payments of medical expenses for Mark's grandchildren are not subject to gift or GST tax.

Employment for an Heir

If you're very charitably inclined, have the financial wherewithal to make substantial gifts, and have specific charitable goals you would like to meet, a private foundation may be an ideal planning technique for you. With the exercise of caution and reason, in some instances, it is feasible to have your private foundation employ family members in the process of operating the foundation and making grants to appropriate charities, including the Society and other specific MS research projects. This can provide your children or other heirs with the following benefits:

- Training in philanthropy to help them better understand their obligations to society and how to deal with the wealth you anticipate them to eventually inherit.
- The foundation board may include outside experts active in fields of MS research and programming to help guide your heirs in the optimal support of projects to benefit MS research or other issues.
- The responsibility, pride, and confidence of being actively engaged in responsible charitable endeavors.
- Compensation commensurate with the services they provide, their skills and abilities, and so on.
- The ability to control family wealth that you contribute to the foundation and for which you receive an income tax deduction, for many years in the future. Because a foundation is only required to distribute 5% of its assets for charitable purposes each year, the large donations you contribute could continue to grow even while annual donations are distributed, as long as your foundation realizes more than 5% return on its investments.

A private foundation is a private charity. Because it is not "public," the tax laws impose a host of specific requirements that must be met. Failure to meet these requirements can cause substantial tax costs and penalties. If the compensation paid to your heirs is not reasonable, it could be viewed as an act of self-dealing, and a penalty tax could be imposed. If the excessive or inappropriate compensation is not refunded, the tax could be 200% of the amount paid. You should also be aware that the tax form filed by your foundation, Form 990-PF, is a public document that can be identified by anyone. If, subject to these and other limitations and caveats, you are comfortable with the approach, a private foundation can provide reasonable compensation and employment for your heirs.

Donating Without Diminishing an Heir's Inheritance

Insurance Can Be Used to Replace Assets Donated

You might be willing to make a substantial contribution to the Society, but are concerned about the impact the contribution will have on your heirs. In many instances, you might be satisfied to address this concern by combining a life insurance plan with your charitable donation. This is often done whether the donation to the Society is outright, in a charitable remainder trust (CRT), or uses some other technique. Insurance planning is frequently combined with charitable planning to replace the value of the property donated to the charity with insurance passing to your heirs. In fact, this approach is so common that the trust often used to hold life insurance intended to replace the assets you donate to the Society is called a wealth replacement trust. It replaces the wealth you've given to the organization through other techniques.

Insurance Planning and Your Charitable Remainder Trust

This concept is often used when you make a donation to the Society using a CRT because the CRT provides you the cash flow to buy insurance to replace the assets donated. The CRT technique was illustrated in several earlier examples; here, the focus is on coordinating the CRT with insurance so that your heirs still receive a significant inheritance, even though you made a large gift. You fund a CRT with appreciated assets and receive an income stream back. You then use some portion of the increased income stream to establish and fund an irrevocable life insurance trust (ILIT) for the benefit of your heirs (e.g., your children). You can meet your desired charitable goals of providing for a favored cause, such as the Society. The income tax savings from the charitable contribution deduction provides cash flow to make gifts to an irrevocable life insurance trust, or to your heirs directly, to purchase insurance on your life. The trustee of the ILIT purchases insurance on your life (or, if you are married, second-to-die life insurance on the lives of both you and your spouse) in an amount sufficient to replace the value of the assets that you donated to the Society or to a charitable remainder trust designed to benefit the organization.

⊕ E X A M P L E : Sheila Green donates real estate to a CRT that will eventually benefit the Society. She will avoid a substantial capital gains tax when the CRT sells the property. The proceeds will be invested, and Sheila will receive an annual income. Sheila will use some of this cash flow from the CRT to make annual gifts to an ILIT. The trustee of the trust will use the proceeds to buy life insurance on Sheila's life, sufficient to replace some portion or all of the value of the donated property to Sheila's son and daughter after her death. The children will receive the same $1 million on Sheila's death that they would have received had the planning not been undertaken. However, had there been no planning, the real estate that the children would have received may have been reduced by a 50% marginal estate tax, transfer costs, and more. Thus, the children may actually receive more than double the net value with the charitable/insurance plan than without it.

⊕ E X A M P L E : Frank Barker, age 65, owns non–income producing property worth $1 million, which he purchased for $200,000. Giving the property to a CRT could generate a $417,000 contribution deduction. This could provide an income tax savings of approximately $140,000. Furthermore, Frank will avoid approximately $220,000 capital gains on the sale of the property. With no further planning, the property would have been included in Frank's estate, generating a $500,000 state and federal estate tax. The CRT will pay Frank

$60,000 per year for his life. Frank can make annual gifts to his son, daughter-in-law, and two grandchildren (or to a different trust designed to own insurance) totaling $48,000, using the annual gift tax exclusion (he can gift up to $12,000 to any number of people each year with no gift tax consequence). This amount can be used by the children to purchase $1 million in life insurance on Frank's life, sufficient to replace the $1 million property given to the CRT for the Society. Frank's heirs will receive the same $1 million on his death that they would have received had the planning not been undertaken.

Using Life Insurance to Protect a Charitable Remainder Trust's Cash Flow

The previous discussion showed how you can use life insurance to replace the value of assets you donate to the Society directly, or to a CRT to benefit the organization. Another financial risk exists. A key financial benefit of a CRT is the periodic cash flow (annuity or uni-trust) that you, as the life or income beneficiary of the CRT, receive for life or for a specific period of years. Implicit in this planning is the idea that you will survive long enough to receive sufficient distributions to make the plan viable. If you die prematurely, you'll have received few distributions. Furthermore, if you have children or others who depend on you financially (e.g., a daughter with MS), and who are not beneficiaries of the CRT, your death will terminate the cash flow distribution they were indirectly depending on. This risk is one you might be able to address with an insurance plan. In the appropriate circumstances, the charitable remainder technique can be combined with a life insurance policy on the life of income or life-beneficiary of the CRT. If you die prematurely, the insurance proceeds can supplement the income stream that your family will have lost. This could be done, for example, with a life insurance trust for the benefit of your spouse and/or children. The life insurance trust should be structured to ensure that the proceeds are not included in your taxable estate. In some cases, an insurance arrangement providing for decreasing coverage (to approximate the decline in the loss of expected income as you live through the intended term of the trust) can be used.

Using Charitable Giving to Teach Your Heirs the Value of Charitable Giving

Estate planning should not be only about the transmission of wealth: It should be about the transmission of values, particularly philanthropy, to your heirs. A host of ways are available for you to accomplish this lofty goal—a goal that can provide considerable benefit to your heirs. Consider the following:

- Establish trusts under your will that direct your heirs to distribute some specified amount or percentage of the trust each year to charities. You could provide guidance about how this should be done and select at least one of the trustees who has the skills and personality to help inculcate charitable values and guide your heirs in these endeavors.

- Set up a private foundation and actively involve your heirs in serving on the board of directors to allocate charitable grants.
- Make a donation to a donor-advised fund (DAF) and designate your heirs in the DAF agreement as the people responsible for making the decisions about which charitable causes should be benefited.
- Establish a charitable lead trust (CLT) and have the funds which are required to be distributed each year allocated at the direction of your heirs.

You can set up guidelines, even quite specific ones, within any of these documents designating how, when, and for what purposes charitable gifts should be dispersed. For example, if you want to benefit the Society, or certain specific types of programs, you can provide parameters that guide your donations, but leave the details to your heirs.

Chapter Summary

This chapter has provided a review of many donors' common goals that can be met as part of an overall charitable, financial, and estate plan. Charitable planning is not only about maximizing your tax deductions. It can be about a myriad of personal and financial goals ranging from inculcating charitable giving values in your heirs, to maximizing your cash flow, to creating a retirement plan, and more. Flexible and creative planning can help you achieve many goals and encourage and facilitate even greater donations.

CHAPTER SIX

TAX RULES
FOR
CHARITABLE GIVING

A HOST OF TECHNICAL TAX RULES affect your donations to the National Multiple Sclerosis Society (the Society) and the amount of tax benefit you'll receive. Although we have intentionally tried to minimize discussions of these many technical rules—focusing instead on planning ideas to help you achieve your charitable and personal goals—this chapter is the exception. Here, we'll overview many significant tax rules. Although it is assumed that you'll rely on your advisers (primarily your accountant) to deal with the more complex matters, a basic understanding of tax laws, as they pertain to charitable giving, will help you discuss knowledgeably with your accountant the charitable plan you wish to implement.

Income Tax Planning

Your donation to the Society will, in most cases, provide some type of income tax benefit. For many donations, maximizing your income tax charitable contribution deductions will be a key part of the planning. The following discussions review some of the many rules that will affect your deduction. (Be advised that a host of exceptions and nuances exist for every rule discussed; these are the province of your tax advisor and well beyond the scope of this book. Don't attempt to undertake charitable planning without expert advice.)

Income Tax Deductions for Your Donations to the Society

General Requirements to Qualify for a Contribution Deduction: Charitable contributions are deducted on your personal income tax return as an itemized deduction on Schedule A, Form 1040. To be deductible, contributions must be gifts to, or for the use of, a qualified charitable organization, which includes the National Multiple Sclerosis Society. You, as the donor, must part with something of value, and the Society as the donee/charity, must receive something of value. Generally, you cannot receive anything of value back from the Society for having made the donation, and you must donate the entire interest in the property (see below). The Society must be given full control over the cash or property you donate, and you must intend to benefit the organization in order for you to receive a tax deduction. This does not mean you cannot specify a particular use of the funds, but the Society—not a particular individual—must benefit. While this should not prove restrictive for anyone looking to benefit common goals of the Society, it would prevent you from using the organization to channel funds to a particular individual you are looking to help.

✸ EXAMPLE: Joseph Smith was touched by a single mother who lost her job as an executive secretary because her employer didn't understand or accommodate the impact her MS had on her ability to perform her duties. She lost her health insurance and was in severe financial need. Joseph donated

$10,000 to the Society to provide assistance to this particular woman. Although Joseph's cause and intent are admirable, he cannot use the Society as a conduit to benefit a particular individual, however great the need. Joseph could donate the funds to the Society with the direction that they use the donation to fund programs that would help people in similar situations, even if this particular person also benefits. The donation must be placed in the control of the Society.

✪ EXAMPLE: Gary Lane has been a regular and substantial contributor to the Society. Gary's interests were particularly piqued by a discussion he had with an investigator researching communications between oligodendrocyte, myelin, axons, astrocytes, and Schwann cells. The investigator is researching why axonal damage does not occur at the nodes of Ranvier if the axons are exposed in that area. Gary can make a donation to the Society and direct that it be used to further this particular investigator's work, but he cannot use the organization as a conduit to benefit an individual recipient, even a researcher.

As illustrated throughout this book, most of the general tax rules affecting charitable contributions are replete with exceptions, exclusions, and special rules. Many of these are quite complex, and often they are not intuitive, which is why it's advisable to review the details of every charitable plan of significance with your accountant.

Donor Receives Benefit: If you realize any benefit from the property donated to the Society, the amount of the charitable contribution deduction must be reduced by the value of the benefit you received. You are generally allowed to rely on an estimate of the value of any benefit provided to you by the Society. Goods or services provided to you as a donor can be ignored if they are of insubstantial value. The IRS views donor benefits as insubstantial if either:

- The donation you make is $89 or more (inflation adjusted) and the benefits you receive don't exceed 2% of the donation; or
- Your contribution is $44.50 or greater (inflation adjusted), and the only benefits are token items such as T-shirts or other items bearing the Society's name that have a wholsale value of less than $8.90 (inflation adjusted).

⚙ E X A M P L E : Linda Worth attended a Society gala dinner. The cost of a ticket is $300. She receives a gift bag of items, each of which costs the Society $8.90 or less. Linda's contribution will not be reduced by the value of these token gift items, although it will be reduced by the cost of the dinner itself, of which the Society will advise her.

⊛ EXAMPLE: Helen Wall donated $500 to an event at her local Society chapter in order to be listed as a sponsor in the event advertisements. She also received a special jacket worth $95 for becoming a sponsor. Helen's $500 donation does not have to be reduced by the intangible benefit she might receive by being listed as a sponsor in the advertising, but she does have to reduce her deduction by the $95 value of the jacket since its value is more than 2% of her donation, and the cost to the Society exceeds $8.90.

Value of Your Contribution Deduction: The higher your marginal income tax bracket, the greater the income tax benefits of charitable giving. The tax benefits of charitable giving can be illustrated with a simple example:

⊛ EXAMPLE: Fiona Smith donates $1,000 to the Society. Fiona lives in a state that has a state income tax. Fiona's marginal federal income tax bracket is 33%, and her marginal state income tax bracket is 3.5%. The effective tax benefit is $353.45, calculated as follows: [(state tax benefit is $1,000 × 3.5% = $35) + (federal tax benefit is $1,000 × 33% = $330 – {$35 state tax benefit × 33% federal rate = $11.55})]. Thus, the actual out-of-pocket cost of the donation is $646.55 [$1,000 – $353.45]. If Fiona's marginal federal income tax bracket is 39.6%, and her marginal state income tax bracket is 3.5%, the effective tax benefit is [(state income tax benefit is $1,000 × 3.5% = $35) + (federal tax benefit $396 − {$35 state tax benefit × 39.6% federal rate = $13.86})] = $409.86. Thus, the actual out-of-pocket cost of the donation is $590.14 [$1,000 − $409.86]. If Fiona is subject to the Alternative Minimum Tax (AMT), the AMT rate would instead apply.

Amount Deductible: When you make a cash contribution of property to or for the use of a qualified charitable organization such as the Society, the amount of the cash payment, subject to the percentage limitation rules described below, is deductible, unless you receive something of value in return. If you donate property to the Society, the fair market value of the property, subject to the percentage limitations and other requirements outlined below, is generally deductible.

Contribution of Property That Has Declined in Value: Donations of property that has declined in value are generally not advisable because no loss deduction will be available for the difference between the fair market value of the property and the adjusted basis of the property. Instead, you will achieve a better income tax result by selling the property and donating the net proceeds. This will permit you to deduct the loss, and then claim a charitable deduction for the cash donated.

Contribution of Property That Has Appreciated: If the value of the donated property exceeds your adjusted tax basis (what you paid to purchase the property, plus improvements, less depreciation) in the property, additional limitations and adjustments may apply depending on the type of property (e.g., real property, personal property, etc.). These limitations are discussed in both Chapter 4 and this chapter.

Capital Gain Property: Generally, if you donate appreciated capital gain property, you will be entitled to deduct the full fair market value of the donated property. Capital gain property is property that, had it been sold instead of being donated to the charity, would have generated capital gain. However, if you deduct the entire fair market value of the property (thus avoiding tax on the appreciation if the Alternative Minimum Tax does not apply), the amount of the charitable deduction is limited to 30% of your adjusted gross income (AGI). This income limitation is explained in greater detail below.

Special Election to Avoid 30% Limitation on Deduction of Appreciated Property Donation: You can avoid the above rule limiting your contribution deduction to 30% of your adjusted gross income (AGI) if you instead agree to reduce the fair market value of the donated property by any appreciation in claiming your tax deduction. If this is done, you can then claim a deduction of up to 50% of your AGI. If the 30% limitation will apply to you, and you don't have substantial appreciation in the asset involved, this election can be beneficial.

✿ EXAMPLE: Sandra Johnson is a real estate investor. She purchased a single tract of land that she believed would appreciate when a county road project was completed. She has done nothing to improve the land. She purchased this particular lot five years earlier for $250,000. If she sold the lot she, as a passive investor, would realize capital gains income. She donates the lot to the Society to use for additional parking at a regional MS center. The lot is presently valued at $320,000. Her charitable contribution deduction is $320,000. However, the amount Sandra can deduct is limited to 30% of her adjusted gross income. If, instead, Sandra attached a signed statement to her income tax return (an election in tax parlance) stating that she will limit her deduction by reducing the fair value of the property ($320,000) by the appreciation ($70,000) so that her deduction will be only $250,000 (which is her adjusted tax basis), the 30% AGI limitation will not apply.

Ordinary Income Property: If the property you donate to the Society had instead been sold, if that sale would have generated ordinary income or short-term capital gain, then your charitable contribution deduction is limited to the fair market value of the property, reduced by the ordinary income or short-term capital gain portion. This will often be what you paid for the property.

✿ E X A M P L E : Mary Rhodes is a real estate developer. She purchases tracts of land, subdivides them, installs roads, sewers, and other improvements, and then sells developable lots to future homeowners. Mary is a dealer in real estate. She has a lot that she purchased five months earlier for $250,000, which she held for sale in the ordinary course of her business. If she sold the lot she, as a dealer, would realize ordinary income. She donates the lot to the Society to use for additional parking at a regional MS center. The lot is presently valued at $320,000. Her charitable contribution deduction is limited to her $250,000 adjusted tax basis. If Mary had instead sold the lot, she would have paid a 40% combined federal and state income tax, since capital gains treatment is not available.

Part Gift/Part Sale of Property to the Society

You might like the idea of donating appreciated assets to the Society to support the organization and realize a significant income tax benefit. However, you might not be in a financial position to donate the entire asset. You might wish to receive some cash for a portion of the value of the property donated, if the value of the property is greater than the amount the donor is willing to donate. This arrangement is referred to as a bargain sale. In many cases, prospective donors find the sale of their property to the Society for an amount equal to their tax basis or cost an acceptable arrangement. You would thus only be donating the appreciation in your property. This provides a psychological effect of not really parting with principal—just giving away appreciation.

If you consummate a bargain sale (part sale/part gift), the easiest way to understand the transaction is to view it as if it were two independent transactions.

> ✪ EXAMPLE: Katy Cowen owns investment land that would be ideally suited for the construction of a new MS facility in her area. She is willing to donate the $2 million property but, after consulting with her financial planner, determines that she needs $500,000 to ensure her retirement income goals. Katy purchased the property for $220,000 many years ago. Katy offers the Society the purchase of the property for $500,000, which is one-quarter of the actual value. For tax purposes, it's as if Katy sold one-quarter of the property to the Society for $500,000 and donated three-quarters of the property with a fair market value of $1,500,000. The tax basis of the property must be allocated to each component. Katy's $220,000 tax basis allocable to the sale component can be calculated by applying the following formula: [Amount Realized on Sale/Total Fair Market Value × Adjusted Tax Basis] [$500,000/$2,000,000 × $220,000] = $55,000. The gain on the sale component is: [Amount Realized on Sale − Allocable Adjusted Tax Basis] [$500,000 − $55,000] = $445,000.

Percentage Limitations on Your Charitable Contributions

Charitable contribution deductions are limited to specified percentages of your Adjusted Gross Income (AGI). When planning large contributions, these limits must be carefully considered by your accountant. These are complex, technical and exceedingly boring. You'll never have to be an expert in these, but an overall awareness of what the rules are about will help you get through a charitable planning meeting with your tax adviser with a better understanding of some important restrictions on your donations.

Definition of Adjusted Gross Income: The percentage limitations are all pegged to a percentage of your AGI, which is defined as all of your gross receipts (income) less certain deductions allowed under Code Section 62.

50% Limitation: There are really two 50% limitations that apply to your donations:

- First, all your donations in aggregate (i.e., those to the National Multiple Sclerosis Society and all other charities) cannot exceed 50% of your AGI.
- Second, your contributions (excluding capital gain property) to those charitable organizations characterized as 50% limit organizations cannot exceed 50% of your AGI. This includes public charities such as the Society, certain private operating foundations,

private non-operating foundations that make qualifying distributions of 100% of the contributions they receive within 2 1/2 months following the close of the tax year, and certain private foundations whose contributions are pooled in a common fund and the earnings of which are then paid to public charities.

If your contributions in any year exceed the limitations you can deduct them in any of the next five years, if this limit doesn't prevent their deduction in those years. This is called a carry over.

30% Limitation: There are really two 30% limitations that apply to your donations:

- Deductions for your contributions to certain charities that don't qualify as 50% charities (defined above) are limited the 30% of your AGI. This includes contributions to veteran organizations, fraternal societies, and certain private foundations.
- Contributions for the use of a charity are also subject to this limit. This includes, for example, a donation of an income interest in property.
- Contributions of capital gain property (when you claim a deduction for the fair market value of the property) to 50% limit organizations are limited. This occurs if you do not make the special election to reduce the contribution by the amount of appreciation, as discussed earlier in this chapter.

20% Limitation: Contributions of capital gain property to organizations that do not qualify as 50% limit organizations are limited to 20% of your AGI. These are generally donations to family private foundations. This restriction does not apply to gifts to the Society, but may affect your overall planning.

Calculating the Deduction Limitation: If your contributions are subject to the percentage limitations summarized above, you'll have to use the following ordering rules to determine how those limitations apply. Thus, even if some of the above percentage restrictions don't apply to your donations to the Society, they may affect your overall tax results.

- First, consider gifts to organizations that qualify for the 50% limitation.
- Next, consider contributions that are subject to the 30% limitation on non-capital gain property donated to charities that are not 50% deduction charities, and donations for the use of a charity. This tier is subject to two limitations. First, all the donations in this category must be limited to 30% of your AGI. Once that is calculated, the deductions as limited cannot exceed 50% of your AGI, reduced by all 50% contributions in the preceding paragraph.
- Next, the 30% limitation on capital gain property is applied. Once that is calculated, the deductions as limited cannot exceed 50% of your AGI, reduced by all 50% contributions in the earlier paragraph.

- Then, you can consider donations subject to the 20% limitation. Again, these are donations of capital gain assets to non–50% charities. These donations are limited to 20% of your AGI. The deduction so calculated cannot exceed 30% of your AGI, reduced by the 30% of AGI contributions above. Then the deductions as limited by all these calculations cannot exceed 50% of your AGI, reduced by all 50% contributions in the earlier paragraph. Each of the percentages limitations is thus applied in a pyramid effect to the lower-tier limitations.
- The excess of your contributions in the current year over these various limitations can be deducted in (is carried over to) the next five years subject to the same 20%, 30%, and 50% limitations.
- Contributions to veterans' organizations, non-profit cemetery organizations, and fraternal societies subject to the 20% limit may not be carried over to future years. So, if you made these types of contributions, as well as a large donation to the Society, if your donation to the organization pushes you beyond 20% of your AGI, you might lose the tax benefit of otherwise deductible contributions.

    ☞ E X A M P L E : Janet Williams has adjusted gross income of $50,000 and resides in a state without an income tax. She donates $2,000 by check to a public charity. She also donates land with a fair market value of $30,000 to the Society. She had paid $10,000 (adjusted tax basis) for the land. Janet donated

$5,000 to a private foundation (a 30% limit organization). The following AGI limitations must be considered: Janet's 50% limit is $25,000; Janet's 30% limit is $15,000; and Janet's 20% limit is only $10,000. The result of these limitations is as follows: The cash contribution of $2,000 is allowed first. The contribution of the land is limited to 30% of the Janet's AGI, or $15,000. This generates a carryover to future years of $15,000 [$30,000 – $15,000]. The $5,000 contribution to the private foundation is carried over to each of the next five years until used.

Itemized Deduction Rules May Limit Your Contribution Deduction

Standard Deduction: You're entitled to claim certain deductions on your personal tax return for medical expense, tax payments, investment expenses, and so on. These deductions are collectively called itemized deductions. The majority of taxpayers don't itemize deductions because of a tax rule that lets everyone choose to deduct a set amount without any details or substantiation. This set amount, called the standard deduction, simplifies tax reporting for millions of taxpayers. The standard deduction in 2007 for married taxpayers filing a joint income tax return is $10,700. For a single individual, it is $5,350. These amounts increase each year by an inflation adjustment. If your total deductions, including charitable contributions to the Society, are less than the standard deduction, you may not realize any income tax benefit from your donation.

Most wealthy taxpayers claim itemized deductions. These are subject, of course, to limitations that may be imposed by the AMT. If you itemize deductions, you might realize a full income tax benefit for the donations you make to the Society. This was illustrated earlier in this chapter in an example showing the economic value of a tax deduction. However, you're not out of the tax woods just yet. A limitation exists that may affect wealthy taxpayers and reduce the deductions, including charitable contributions that would otherwise qualify as an itemized deduction.

Phase-out of Itemized Deductions: In addition to the gross income percentage limitations discussed above, your charitable contribution deductions may be further reduced as a result of a phase-out of itemized deductions. For income tax purposes, a charitable contribution deduction is part of your overall itemized deductions. Itemized deductions are reduced for tax years 2007 through 2009 by a percentage of your adjusted gross income. This phase-out is complex, and perhaps the only way to determine if it will adversely affect your contributions is to have your accountant prepare a projection of what your tax results are anticipated to be. Your itemized deductions, including contributions to the Society, are limited or reduced by the smaller of the following:

- Two percent of the excess of your AGI over a base amount, which is $156,400 in 2007 for a married couple filing a joint return. The base amount varies by year and tax filing status.
- Eighty percent of the itemized deductions you would otherwise be allowed to deduct.

Paperwork: What Documentation You Need; What You Must Report to the IRS

Paperwork is something no donor wants to deal with, but you have no choice if you want to ensure your tax benefits. The Society and your accountant can help you meet the necessary requirements, so don't be deterred by them. To make the process easier for you, the following discussion is intended to help you understand some of the reporting requirements.

Documenting Cash Donated to the Society

If you donate cash to the Society, your cancelled check (and presumably credit card receipt, if you paid by credit card) will support your contribution deduction. Even for small cash donations, you must have a receipt from the Society, and/or a bank record of the contribution (cancelled check).

> ✪ EXAMPLE: Jeff Johnson participated in a recent Society MS Walk. If he donated $100 by check mailed to his local chapter before the walk, his cancelled check will support his income tax charitable contribution deduction. However, if Jeff donated an additional $20 in cash at the walk itself, he must obtain and save a receipt from the Society to claim a tax deduction.

For cash contributions in excess of $250 or more, the Society will report your contributions to the IRS. If you make a contribution in excess of $75, where part of the payment is a contribution and part is for goods or services, a written statement containing a good faith estimate of the deductible portion will be provided to you. Save that letter with your tax records for the year.

⚙ EXAMPLE: Janet Wilson attended a Society fund raising dinner for a cost of $300 per ticket. The actual value of the dinner served was $54. The Society must give Janet a written notice that only $246 is deductible.

Documenting Marketable Securities Donated to the Society

If you donate publicly traded marketable securities, no appraisal is required. If you donate securities that are not publicly traded, an appraisal is required only if the claimed market value of the contribution is greater than $10,000.

Documenting Property Donated to the Society

The IRS is clearly concerned that taxpayers have abused the right to donate property (car, art, etc.) to charities and claim a tax deduction. These rules should not dissuade you from making such donations to the Society, but rather encourage you to plan such gifts carefully with your accountant so that you meet the necessary requirements. The documentation you'll need to support your tax deduction increases with the value of the donation you are making. Where donations of two or more similar properties are made in the same tax year, they will be aggregated for purposes of applying these tests.

Over $500, Less Than $5,000: For property donations, a reliable written record and a receipt from the Society setting forth its name and other pertinent facts, such as the date and location of the contribution, is required. You'll have to provide the IRS with a detailed description of the property, the approximate date the property was acquired (if you constructed the property, the date the property was substantially completed), an explanation of how you acquired the property (gift, purchase, exchange, etc.), the fair market value of the property on the date of the donation, and a description of the method used to determine the fair market value of the property. Your accountant will have to file Form 8283, "Noncash Charitable Contributions" with your tax return.

Over $5,000, Less Than $500,000: If the value of the property contributed is greater than $5,000, the IRS requires that you obtain a qualified appraisal and file it with your income tax return.

Over $500,000: The IRS may require additional reporting. Your accountant can guide you.

If the property you donated to the Society was a car, boat, or airplane, additional documentation rules apply to confirm whether the organization made significant use of the property, made major repairs, or simply sold it. The IRS has sought to crack down on taxpayers donating these items and claiming deductions for values much larger than the amounts the charity receiving the property sold it for. Again, these reporting requirements should not dissuade you from donating property; they should simply motivate you to have your accountant corroborate that you have the necessary documentation.

If you're a partner in a partnership or a shareholder in an S corporation that makes a property donation to the Society, the partnership or S corporation must comply with these requirements. If it doesn't, you'll lose the deduction that was passed through to you to report on your personal tax return. A partnership or S corporation must also file Form 8283 if it makes a property donation to the Society. A copy of the form must be provided to each partner or shareholder who receives an allocation of the deduction. Make sure that the entity accountant complies with the necessary reporting requirements.

Documenting Non-Cash Donations: Appraisal Rules

You may need to meet a number of requirements for appraisals. As with all documentation rules, these should not deter you from making property donations; rather, they should encourage you to have your accountant shepherd the process along to be sure all the technicalities are handled properly.

An appraisal is necessary, as noted earlier, for many types of property donations to the Society. In many cases, you will have to obtain a qualified appraisal, made within a certain time, to be certain that it reflects the value at the time of your donation (not more than 60 days prior to the donation, or later than the due date of your income tax return). To be a qualified appraiser, the appraiser must be a regularly practicing and paid professional (not Uncle Joe) who has not been barred from practicing before the IRS. The appraiser's compensation cannot be set as a percentage of the appraised value. The appraisal may not be provided by the Society or the person who sold the property to you.

Penalties can be assessed if the value of donated property is overstated. The penalty is charged at a 40% rate if the amount claimed on your tax return as a deduction (the fair market value of the property or the adjusted basis) is more than 200% of the correct amount.

You cannot deduct the cost of obtaining the appraisal as a charitable contribution. The cost can be deducted as a miscellaneous itemized deduction on Schedule A, Form 1040, to the extent all miscellaneous deductions exceed 2% of your adjusted gross income. This rule will make it unlikely that you will realize a deduction for the cost of the appraisal.

Charitable Remainder Trusts

Charitable remainder trusts (CRTs) were illustrated in a several examples in prior chapters. Those illustrations focused on a specific application of CRTs in the context of the examples used and did not provide an overview of CRTs. The following discussion will provide that overview, to help you gain a better understanding of the technique

Requirements for CRT: A number of requirements must be met for a CRT to qualify for favorable tax benefits. The legal document (trust) that creates the CRT must state that the trust cannot be changed (irrevocable). The payment made from the CRT to you (and any other current recipients) must be for a term of years not in excess of 20 years, or for the lives of the individual beneficiaries named (e.g., you and your spouse). The yearly payment percentage must be equal to at least 5% of the net fair market value of the trust assets. The CRT cannot have a payout of greater than 50% of the fair market value of its assets. The anticipated value of the assets in the CRT when the term ends (after the specified number of years, or the death of the persons named to receive payments), which will be received by the Society (the remainder interest), determined on the date the property is contributed to the CRT, must be at least 10% of the value of the property.

> ✪ E X A M P L E : Lisa and Stanley Clark want to establish a CRT. Although they want to benefit the Society, they are also concerned with receiving a significant annual cash flow (annuity) to support them during retirement. If the CRT is established to pay 8% per year, and Lisa and Stanley are ages 55 and 54, respectively (and assuming the applicable IRS interest rate for

the calculation is 5.8%), the CRT won't meet the 10% test. Effectively, the Society would be expected to get nothing when the trust terminates, based on the high 8% payout and the young ages of the two donors. If Lisa and Stanley instead reduce the payout to them to 5.5%, on a $1 million donation to the CRT, they will receive $55,000 annually for the remainder of their lives. On the death of the last of Lisa or Stanley, the Society will be expected to receive $232,844. The 10% test is met, and the CRT will qualify for tax purposes. Lisa and Stanley will be able to deduct that amount as a charitable contribution deduction on their personal income tax returns.

Types of Charitable Remainder Trusts. There are different types of CRTs, each appropriate for different donor circumstances. Many of these have been illustrated in preceding chapters. The variations in CRTs permit flexibility to use CRTs to meet a variety of donor goals:

- Charitable remainder annuity trusts (CRATs) provide you (or people you designate) with a fixed annuity, as the current beneficiaries. Typically, the donor and the donor's spouse are named beneficiaries. However, if you wanted to name another person, such as a loved one with MS, in order to supplement their income, that could be done. However, the possibility of a gift tax must to be planned for. The minimum payout rate from the CRAT to the donor and other named beneficiaries cannot be less than 5%. The payments to the beneficiaries are calculated based on the fair market value of the property when it is first transferred to the CRAT. Once the trust is established, no further contributions can be made to it. If the trust income is insufficient to meet the required annual return, principal must be invaded. No further additions may be made to a CRAT once it is set up.

- Charitable remainder uni-trusts (CRUTs) provide a form of variable annuity benefit to the current beneficiaries. The minimum rate of return to the income beneficiaries is 5%. However, unlike the CRAT, this payment is calculated based on the fair market value of the property determined on an annual basis. Thus, if the assets held by the CRUT increase in value over time, which is anticipated, a uni-trust payment will grow over time. This contrasts with the payments under a CRAT, which are fixed. Thus, for a younger donor, a CRUT provides an inflation hedge to the periodic payments. The annual determination of a payment for a CRUT requires an annual appraisal, which for any property that is difficult to value (e.g., closely held business interests and real estate), could be expensive. The CRUT may provide that, if the annual income earned by the trust property is insufficient to meet the required distribution to the income beneficiaries, principal may be invaded. If principal is not required to be invaded, then the trust must provide that the deficit will be made up in later years. Once a CRT in the form of a uni-trust is established, additional contributions may be made in later years, under certain conditions.
- Income-only uni-trusts (NI-CRUTs) are a modified form of the CRUT. A NI-CRUT can be planned so that the current beneficiary receives an income-only arrangement. In a NI-

CRUT, the current beneficiary would only receive the actual trust income if the income is less than the fixed percentage payment required (e.g., 5% of the trust's principal). A NI-CRUT should include its own definition of how income is to be calculated to avoid having your state laws (Principal and Income Act) unintentionally impact your planning.

> ❂ EXAMPLE: Thomas McDonald established a NI-CRUT to benefit the Society. He contributed $1 million to the trust, but the trust is invested only in growth stocks. The actual income earned by the NI-CRUT in the prior year was only $10,000. Even though the trust document requires a $50,000 distribution (5% × $1 million), the trust will only distribute $10,000 to Thomas.

- Net Income with a make-up uni-trusts (NIM-CRUTs) are a modified form of the NI-CRUT. A NIM-CRUT can be planned, like the NI-CRUT, so that you (as the current beneficiary) receive an income-only arrangement. But the distinguishing feature of a NIM-CRUT is that it includes a make-up provision. In early years, actual income may be substantially less than the 5% required CRUT payment. In later years, sufficient income may be earned to pay not only that year's payment, but to make up for some of the payments not paid in prior years. These rules were used in earlier examples that illustrated how a CRT can be planned to effectively function as a retirement plan.

✪ EXAMPLE: Daphne Hanson owns raw land worth $500,000. This land produces very modest income from an occasional rental for overflow parking to a nearby catering hall. Daphne donates this property to a NIM-CRUT that will eventually benefit the Society. Until the property is sold and cash is made available for income-producing investments, or the property is developed to generate significant rental income, there may be little or no income. In later years, after the property is sold or made productive, when the net income of the trust exceeds the specified percentage of trust assets required to be paid (e.g., 5%), this excess can then be paid to Daphne—as the income beneficiary—to make up for the shortfall in prior years. The shortfall is determined based on the difference between the amounts actually paid in prior years, the occasional and nominal rent, and the amounts that were required to have been paid based on the fixed percentage, or $25,000 per year.

- Flip charitable remainder uni-trusts (FLIP CRUTs) are another variation on the CRUT that provide additional planning opportunities and flexibility. In a FLIP-CRUT, you would be paid, as in the NI-CRUT, the lesser of the current income of the CRUT or the specified percentage, 5% being the minimum. When a triggering event defined in the trust document occurs, the payment method changes, or "flips" from the lesser of income or the 5% payment, to a fixed percentage. A typical "flip" event is the sale of non–income producing assets, such as growth stocks or raw land.

✪ E X A M P L E : Helen Owens inherited stock in a major company. When her mother bequeathed the stock to her, it was worth a mere $1 per share. It is now worth $100 per share, and pays almost no dividend. Helen wants to save capital gains tax on the sale, benefit the Society, and secure her financial future. Helen believes that, despite her MS, she'll be able to work a few more years, but not many more. When Helen stops working, the stock contributed to the FLIP-CRUT can be sold. Once sold, the trustee can invest the proceeds in income-producing assets and pay Helen a fixed percentage of that amount for the rest of Helen's life. Helen opts to use a FLIP-CRUT because, until the stock is sold, the CRUT won't have any cash flow to pay her an annuity payment.

- Inter-vivos CRTs (of any variety) are established during your lifetime.
- Testamentary CRTs (of any variety) are established in your will or in another legal document and take effect upon your death.

A number of other CRT permutations can further contribute to planning flexibility.

Income Tax Deductions of a CRT Compared to an Out Right Gift of Property. If you donate property directly to the Society, unless any of the special exceptions or rules discussed earlier apply, you will receive an income tax deduction for the full value of the property. However, you cannot receive anything in return, other than the knowledge of having helped an important cause. If, instead, you donate property to a charitable remainder trust (CRT) benefiting the Society, you (and others you name) will receive a periodic payment, possibly for life. The Society will only receive the value of the property (or what it is then invested in) after your death (or the death of you and the other named current beneficiaries) or the CRT term. Therefore, the charitable contribution deduction will be reduced considerably with a CRT, compared to an outright gift. You also need to weigh your desire to contribute currently to the Society efforts. It might be decades before the organization receives actual dollars for programming from your CRT. That is not a reason to limit the use of this type of planning to benefit the Society, but to encourage you to realize that, if you wish to benefit current research and programs, current dollars are needed in addition to CRT deferred dollars.

Income Tax Deduction on Forming a CRT. When you donate property to a CRT, you will be entitled to a deduction for income tax purposes. The deduction is based on the present value of the charitable remainder interest that the Society is expected to receive when your CRT ends. The amount of the charitable contribution deduction is equal to the fair market value of the property at the time of the donation to the CRT, less the present value of the income interest retained by you (or by you and your spouse, or any other named beneficiary). The value of the income tax deduction to you will depend on numerous factors, including your marginal tax bracket (the higher the better—remember, capital gains are presently being taxed at historically low rates), the income interest reserved to you and perhaps others (the greater the income interest, the lower the tax deduction), the applicability of the charitable contribution limitations discussed earlier, and other factors.

Gift and Estate Tax Consequences of a CRT. Although the focus in this section is on income tax planning for your charitable contribution deductions, a brief note on the estate and gift tax implications of your CRT is worthwhile. In addition to the current income tax deduction, you may also receive a valuable estate tax benefit as well. If you are one of the income beneficiaries of the charitable trust, the value of the trust will be included in your gross estate when you die. However, since the interest will pass to a qualified charity (the Society), an offsetting estate tax charitable contribution deduction occurs. Thus, the value of the property donated will be effectively removed from your estate. If anyone is named to receive distributions from the CRT other than you or your spouse (e.g., a child or partner with MS), there will be a gift tax consequence to you when you set up the CRT.

How Beneficiaries Are Taxed on CRT Distributions. The amount paid to a beneficiary (the donor and her spouse) under a CRT retains the character that the property had inside the trust. Some donors mistakenly believe that the only income tax consequence of the CRT is their current income tax deduction, but this is not the full story. The distributions from the CRT have an income tax consequence to you and any other recipients:

- You and the other beneficiaries report a portion of CRT distributions as ordinary income, to the extent of the CRT's current and prior undistributed income.
- After all ordinary income is exhausted, amounts will then be taxed as short-term capital gain, to the extent of current and past undistributed short-term capital gains.
- Next, distributions from the CRT are taxed as long-term capital gain, to the extent of current and past undistributed long-term capital gains.
- Then, distributions are taxed as other income, such as tax exempt income, to the extent of the trust's current and past undistributed income of such character.
- Finally, any further distributions are treated as tax-free distributions of principal.

The trust itself will generally be exempt from tax. Thus, a CRT can sell the appreciated property that you gift to it without incurring any gain (but, as discussed earlier, that gain is recognized by you as distributions are received from the trust). However, if the trust generates unrelated business taxable income (UBTI), it can be subject to tax. This can be an issue when trust assets are debt financed, stock in an active business is contributed to the trust, or other special circumstances occur. These rules are extremely complex and require professional assistance.

Gift Tax Planning

Overview of the Gift Tax

The gift tax is assessed on transfers you make to people during your lifetime. The most common example of gift tax rules, which you are likely to be familiar with, is that you can gift away $12,000 in any year to any person, with no gift tax implications. This is called the gift tax annual exclusion. This amount will be adjusted in future years for inflation. In addition to the gift tax annual exclusion, which you can gift to as many people as you wish, you can gift $1 million in aggregate during your lifetime. After both these amounts are exceeded, a gift tax will apply to tax the value of any assets you give away.

Gift Tax Charitable Contribution Deduction

When you make gifts to charities in excess of the $12,000 per year gift tax exclusion, you will face a gift tax consequence unless the gift is to a qualifying charity, which includes the Society. In such cases, you may qualify for an unlimited gift tax charitable contribution deduction. This amount is inflation indexed.

Using Charitable Lead Trusts to Minimize Gift Tax Consequences

As illustrated in earlier chapters, a charitable lead trust (CLT) can be used in many creative ways to benefit the Society and achieve several important personal goals. This discussion provides a more detailed explanation of the CLT technique.

Overview of CLTs: Although the CLT technique can be used to minimize estate taxes (and can be quite useful in that regard), it is discussed here in the context of minimizing gift taxes on lifetime transfers. A CLT is also called a front trust, because the charitable beneficiary, the Society, receives its income before or in "front" of the ultimate beneficiaries (remainder beneficiaries) receiving their share. Typically, the remainder beneficiaries are your children, although other beneficiaries can be named.

When May a CLT Make Sense for You. The CLT can be a valuable and appropriate estate planning tool when you have (a) charitable intent, (b) the desire to increase the eventual (but not current) net worth of family members or other designated heirs, and (c) the goal of reducing gift and estate taxes. A significant CLT benefit is that appreciation after assets are transferred to the CLT will ultimately pass to your beneficiaries free of any gift or estate tax.

Gift Tax Benefits of a CLT: There are many benefits and reasons for setting up a CLT. CLTs can be significant in reducing gift or estate tax cost. This is especially important in light of the scheduled future increases in the amount you give away estate-tax free (applicable exclusion). It could likely be a pointless waste of money for you to pay a gift tax on a large gift today if the increasing amounts you can give away at death will avoid any estate tax. The reduction in tax cost is achieved by virtue of the fact that the remainder beneficiaries must wait to receive the property until the expiration of the charitable beneficiary's interest. The concept can be illustrated with a simple example.

⚙ EXAMPLE: Ida Jones gives $600,000 to a CLT. The Society will receive annual payments (usually in the form of an annuity or uni-trust amount) for each year of the CLT. The end of the trust will occur after the number of years Ida determined when setting up the trust. Assuming Ida selected a 22-year term for the CLT, Ida's children will receive the trust assets (this will hopefully be substantially more than $600,000, depending on the investment results during the period the Society received payments). If the term of the charitable interest is made long enough, the value of the gift Ida made to his children can be reduced to nearly zero for purposes of the gift tax.

✱ EXAMPLE: Michael Smith gifts $500,000 to a CLT for a 25-year term. The Society is designated as the charity to receive annual payments of $30,000 (at a 6% rate) each year for 25 years. Following the end of the CLT in year 25, Michael's children will receive the trust assets. With a 6% payout and professional investment management, Michael anticipates that the distribution will be substantially more than the $500,000 initial gift. For gift tax purposes, the value of the future gift to Michael's children is reduced from $500,000 to about $100,000. At a 50% estimated tax rate, the gift tax savings could be $200,000 [($500,000 – $100,000) × 50%].

Charitable and Personal Benefits of a CLT: You can meet long-term charitable giving objectives using a CLT. Establishing a CLT will ensure the annual distributions of a specified amount (where an annuity arrangement is used) to the Society for a specified number of years.

✱ EXAMPLE: Wendy Brown has been actively involved with the Society and likes the idea of funding specific projects to ensure their success. She establishes a 20-year CLT for her son, Fred, which will benefit the Society during the interim 20 years. She plans on funding the CLT with $700,000. If the payout rate is 6%, the organization will receive $42,000 per year for 20 years. Wendy arranges an agreement with the Society so that she can approve which projects these funds will be used for. This approach enables Wendy to stay actively involved, provides significant gift tax benefit, and gives the organization assurance that a series of programs in future years will be funded as a result of Wendy's generosity. Wendy can designate in the agreement with the Society that, in the event she resigns, becomes incapacitated, or dies during the CLT term, her son Fred will direct the gifts. Wendy feels that when her son has the maturity and interest, she can resign and enable him to work with the Society on the disbursement of funds so that he can learn more about the organization, philanthropy, and the charitable giving process. Wendy preferred this approach to using a private foundation because she feels she can accomplish the same charitable and educational goals, but will give her son, who lives with MS, an opportunity to be actively involved with the Society and a financial safety net in 20 years. Its Wendy's hope that, if her son has adequate assets when the CLT ends, he'll simply donate the entire trust balance to the Society. Wendy writes a personal letter of instruction to be given to her son when the trust ends to encourage this.

Using a CLT to Time Distributions to Heirs: You can defer and control when your heirs receive funds by timing the termination of the CLT to coincide with different events or milestones (e.g., a beneficiary attaining age 65). This was illustrated in earlier chapters showing how to use a CLT to create a retirement plan for a partner or child. The duration for which a CLT lasts can be coordinated with other estate and financial planning to ensure your children or other heirs the availability of assets for a long-term time horizon.

> ✿ EXAMPLE: Tina Ferguson establishes a trust under her will to pay income annually to her child, Jody, who has MS. Principal is to be paid out of the trust fund in approximately one-third equal amounts when the child attains ages 30, 35, and 40. The child is presently age 22. If Tina establishes a CLT for a duration of 23 years [(40 − 22) + 5], the child will receive the assets of the CLT at age 45. This is timed to continue the five-year payment sequence with the hopes of distributing assets in stages to both protect the remaining assets as well as to minimize the potentially adverse consequences of the child receiving too much wealth at one time in the event that Tina dies prior to her child reaching 45 years of age.

Drawbacks of Using a CLT: Tax and other benefits can only be realized if the CLT meets all applicable tax law requirements, which can be burdensome, costly, and difficult. For example, CLTs can be subject to the rules applicable to private foundations concerning self-dealing, excess business holdings, jeopardy investments, and the like. A special tax is imposed on a CLT that sells or exchanges property within two years after the property was transferred to the CLT. When this rule applies, the CLT is taxed at your income tax rate. The objective of this provision is to prevent you from gaining a tax advantage by transferring property intended for sale to a CLT to sell. CLTs are not tax exempt. A CLT only avoids taxation if the amounts paid to charity are sufficient to offset any income tax otherwise due by the CLT. Gifts to CLTs do not qualify for the gift tax annual exclusion. CLTs create complications for generation-skipping transfer (GST) tax planning. The GST exclusion cannot be allocated to a CLT until the charitable interest ends. Thus, if a 20-year CLAT is used, the GST determination will be made at the end of year 20. If the CLT works as planned, this is when the assets will be highly appreciated and the GST allocation most inefficient to make. The better option is to use a CLUT, because the allocation of the GST amount can be made when you set up the CLT initially. This distinction is complex, but substantial benefits can be achieved with the help of your professional advisors.

Types of CLTs: Your CLT can be prepared in a manner that will qualify it so that all the CLT income is taxed to you (a grantor trust), or so that the CLT pays its own income tax and files its own tax return (a non-grantor trust). In either event, two points warrant your attention. A CLT is never a tax-free entity like the charitable remainder trust discussed in earlier chapters. Because the CLT is not a tax-exempt entity, a deduction will be created each year as the CLT makes its annual donation to the Society. This charitable contribution deduction would be used to offset your income if your CLT is planned as a grantor trust, or the trust's income if it is not. A CLT is usually structured as a non-grantor trust. This means that CLT earnings are not taxed to you. You will not receive an income tax deduction for any charitable contributions made by the CLT during its term. If, instead, the CLT is structured to be a grantor trust, you will be taxed on the income earned by the trust (unless the income is primarily tax-exempt bond income). However, you will also qualify for deductions for the charitable contributions made by the CLT.

Estate Tax Planning

Charitable Bequests Under Your Will: Trusts

Charitable planning can be integrated into your estate planning to accomplish personal, tax, and other goals. You can make direct charitable bequests to the Society in your will. Many people opt to make bequests in their wills, not only to benefit a particular charitable cause, but also to demonstrate to their children and other heirs the importance of making a contribution back to society. You can create trusts to benefit family, or other beneficiaries, who might also benefit charity. Apart from these rather simple approaches that encompass charitable giving, a number of more complex charitable giving techniques use charitable gifts. Many of these were discussed in Chapters 3 through 5, and some are noted again here.

Taxable Versus Probate Estate

Many people confuse the concepts of taxable estate and probate estate. Your taxable estate is comprised of the assets in which you had sufficient interests on your death that the tax laws deem those assets owned by you for purposes of assessing an estate tax. Your probate estate are the assets passing under your will—i.e., through the probate- or court-administered process of administering your estate. Many assets that are not part of your probate estate may still be included in your taxable estate. For example, insurance on your life that you owned, or for which you retained significant rights (incidence of ownership), is not part of your probate estate but is included in your taxable estate. This can be important to understand in planning the magnitude of charitable gifts you wish to provide for in your will or other estate planning documents. Your taxable estate may be much larger than your probate estate, and you may have a greater potential estate tax liability than you anticipate. The distinction between your taxable and probate estate is important if you anticipate giving a certain portion of your estate to the Society.

Estate Tax Charitable Contribution Deduction

Your estate is entitled to deduct any donations made to charity for property included in your estate, if these donations are given to a qualified charity, which includes the National Multiple Sclerosis Society. There are no limitations on the amounts deductible.

Estate Tax Allocation Clause

If your estate must pay estate taxes, those taxes must be paid from some designated portion of your estate. The provision in your will that designates which bequests and which assets are to be used to pay estate taxes is called the tax allocation clause. This provision is too often overlooked or dismissed as standard (boilerplate). That can be a costly mistake that undermines your charitable and other planning. The tax allocation clause should be carefully reviewed with your tax advisors and tailored to meet the specific goals you have for your estate. In most cases, if you make a bequest to the Society, you don't want any portion of that otherwise deductible charitable bequest used toward an estate tax payment. If you do, then the portion of the estate tax paid from the bequest to the Society will reduce that bequest, perhaps undermining your charitable goals. It will also create a spoiler effect in that the dollars used to pay tax would have instead gone to charity, thus reducing your charitable deduction and, in turn, increasing the tax owed. If you have a trust that can benefit both family and the Society, the decision as to how taxes should be allocated is not as clear and professional guidance is essential.

Using Charitable Planning to Minimize Estate Taxes

The charitable lead trust (CLT) discussed earlier, in the context of gift tax planning, can also be used to minimize your estate tax. A testamentary (after your death) CLT can be formed under your will.

�✲ E X A M P L E : Mary Boyle's estate is valued at $4 million. She believes that the estate tax exclusion, presently $2 million, will be increased substantially so that her estate will owe little if any tax. She is reluctant to complicate her life with involved estate tax planning techniques while she is alive, but she isn't fond of the idea of paying a significant tax in the interim. As a "stop-gap" step, she includes a $2 million CLT in her will that effectively eliminates any potential estate tax on the value of her estate in excess of the current $2 million exclusion. If the law changes, she'll only have to delete that bequest in her will, or structure the testamentary CLT so that it is not funded in the event the exclusion amount increases. If it doesn't change, she'll have saved estate tax with no current hassles. If there is an estate tax, the Society will receive the benefit in lieu of the IRS. Mary is rather pleased with the trade-off.

Will You Realize Estate Tax Benefits from Your Donation?

Charitable gifts from your estate can be beneficial from personal and charitable perspectives, regardless of the estate tax benefit. But if your charitable planning is considering the potential benefits of estate tax savings, you must be realistic about what those savings may be.

Properly structured, high-value charitable gifts can significantly reduce potential estate taxes. This can help address potential estate liquidity problems, thus increasing flexibility to retain relatively non-liquid business or real estate interests. The estate tax benefits of charitable giving will similarly depend on your combined federal and state estate tax liability (or just state, if your estate is below the federal exclusion amount, which is $2 million in 2007). If the estate tax continues to phase out (the exclusion is scheduled to increase to $3.5 million in 2009), fewer donors may benefit from federal tax benefits. However, many states have much lower thresholds for estate taxation, and donors in high estate tax states will continue to realize state estate tax benefits for much smaller estates.

Chapter Summary

If any of the techniques discussed in Chapters 1 through 5 of this book interest you, you should review the more detailed rules that affect the techniques in this chapter with your advisors. This chapter discussed many of the more technical aspects of charitable giving, especially the rules for income tax deduction for charitable contributions. The income tax deduction rules are detailed and important, because they will affect how you structure almost any charitable plan to benefit the Society and achieve your other goals. The goal of this chapter was to provide you with a general understanding of some of the important tax issues involved. However, the myriad of exceptions and special rules make it essential that you review these matters with your professional advisers before implementing any plan.

CHAPTER SEVEN

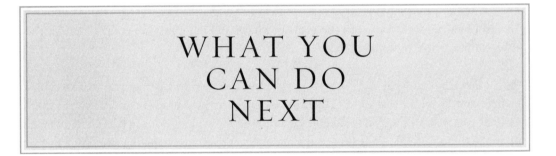

WHAT YOU CAN DO NEXT

Hopefully, you've dog-eared at least a couple of pages containing ideas that caught your attention. The goal of this chapter is to help you turn those dog-ears into action—action that will benefit people and goals you care about. Action that will benefit the National Multiple Sclerosis Society (the Society).

Identify the People, Assets, and Goals You're Concerned About

The first step in your planning process is to identify the people you are concerned about, the assets you have to work with, and the goals you have. No planning can really be undertaken without this essential personal input.

People: Identify all the people in your immediate family, whether you wish to provide for them and, if so, to what extent. Identify any people who are not relatives and the extent to which you wish to provide for them. Background information on each of these people is important to note so that your professional advisers and charitable giving professionals from the Society can work together to make sure these people are provided for. For example, if you have a child who is quite well to do, a charitable lead trust (CLT) that will benefit him in the future may be a great technique. If you have another child who is living with the challenges of MS and unable to work, a trust that will provide benefit in 20 years will be, practically speaking, useless. On the other hand, a charitable remainder trust (CRT) that benefits the latter child immediately, and ensures a quarterly payment for life might be ideal. You must document key details on the people important to you so that your planning can be tailored accordingly. Don't assume that your adviser will know the circumstances of the people important to you. Multiple sclerosis affects everyone differently. You need to openly and clearly communicate details to your advisors. If not, they will make general assumptions, which may not be accurate.

Assets: Prepare (or have your financial planner or accountant prepare or work with you to prepare) a balance sheet listing all assets and liabilities. It is essential for your advisers to understand the assets you have in order to identify the appropriate planning techniques to make those assets best benefit the people you've identified. If your house is a unique beach-front property that has been in your family for generations, a plan that would transfer ownership to the Society, while tax advantageous, might be contrary to one of your key objectives. If your balance sheet reflects liquidity problems, then increasing your liquidity should be a focus of your planning. The assets you own, as well as their specific characteristics and how they fit into your overall financial picture, are all essential facts needed to develop an optimal plan.

Goals: Two people with identical family relationships and assets might have dramatically different plans. The differences are due to the varying goals that people in otherwise similar situations may have. The more clearly and specifically you can elucidate your financial, estate, tax, business, retirement, and personal goals, the better those goals will be achieved. Write them down. Be clear.

Working with Your Advisers

You can't develop, implement, or monitor any charitable giving plan without the coordination of all your advisers. The ideal method of accomplishing this is to have all your key advisers meet to review a proposed plan. While the ideal approach is to have all your advisers at a meeting, this can be impractical because of costs and scheduling. In most cases, the coordination you need between multiple advisers can be accomplished with a few simple conference calls. You might, for example, meet at your attorney's office with a major or planned-gift professional from the Society and make a conference call to your accountant at the appropriate point in the meeting. The key is to involve the necessary advisers and be sure they communicate, so that your plan will be developed in the most advantageous way and, once developed, will be implemented and monitored to ensure your success.

Your advisers could include:

Accountant: You accountant will have to help review and address the income, gift, and estate tax consequences of any plan you are considering. In most cases, it will be advisable for your accountant to complete projections of the anticipated tax result from any plan. These projections can identify traps or opportunities to tailor your plan to better fit your goals. For example, if you're planning a CRT, some strict tests must be met. These requirements should be reviewed in advance of consummating a plan. Once your plan is decided upon, your accountant may have a role in completing financial information, analyzing tax matters, and dealing with other issues. After your plan is implemented, your accountant will have a key role in maintaining and operating your plan. This will include the preparation of any necessary income tax returns.

Financial Planner or Wealth Manager: A key to many of the planning techniques reviewed in this book is investment performance. For example, if you establish a CLT to benefit your child with MS in 20 years, the growth of that portfolio at a rate greater than the payments to the Society during the 20-year term will ensure a substantial retirement plan and safety net. Investment performance must be tailored to the plan. CRTs are tax exempt, CLTs are not. Different plans require different tax sensitivity of investment assets, different rates of return to succeed, and have different cash flow needs.

Insurance Consultant: If you donate large assets directly to the Society, or to a CRT to benefit the Society, you might wish to use insurance to replace the value of the assets your heirs won't receive. If you engage in any type of charitable planning, you might wish to use insurance to protect family or other potential heirs. Insurance is also a powerful charitable giving technique. You can gift a policy you no longer need, have a new policy purchased, or engage in other types of insurance planning to benefit the Society. In all these cases, the input of your insurance consultant to select the optimal insurance product to achieve your goals is vital to the success of your plan. Once your plan is selected, your insurance consultant will be needed to help implement the plan. This may include insurance applications, changing beneficiaries or owners of policies, and other matters. If you gift substantial assets, your need for disability or long-term care insurance may have to be re-evaluated. Once your plan is implemented, your insurance consultant will have to be involved periodically to monitor the plan.

Pension Adviser: If you plan to bequeath retirement assets to the Society, you will need the assistance of your pension adviser.

Attorney: Your attorney must review any legal issues involved in your proposed plan. For example, if your plan involves buying an insurance policy for the Society, your attorney should confirm that the Society has an *insurable interest* so that they can in fact own the policy. An insurable interest means the Society would have the legal right, under state law, to own a policy on your life. Every plan requires that legal documents be drafted. It's not only the specific trust that may be the focal point of your charitable plan, such as a CRT, but all the ancillary documents. If you establish a CRT, your will might include specific provisions relating to that CRT. If you make a bequest in your will of a specific asset to the Society, your attorney will have to draft that language in your will. Your attorney may choose to also modify your durable power of attorney to prevent your agent from making a change or transfer of the asset you've bequeathed to the Society in your will.

Major Gift or Planned-Giving Professional from the Society: If you're planning a significant current or planned gift to the Society, a major or planned-gift professional is an essential part of your planning team. If you're purchasing or donating assets for a gift annuity, you'll need guidance on what is available. If you're funding a specific project or series of projects, the Society professional will help you draft the language of a donor agreement so that your contribution will accomplish the most good. If you want to involve your child or other heir who has MS in the planned-giving process, the Society professional can show you how to accomplish this. Once your plan is conceived, implementation will involve your Society professional coordinating those matters affecting the organization. Once your plan is implemented, depending on the plan, there may be little ongoing Society involvement until the gift or bequest is received. In some instances, however, such as a CLT paying an annuity every year, you'll want ongoing contact with your Society professional.

Develop a Comprehensive Plan

One-dimensional plans don't work. Plans that focus on a single magic bullet or technique don't work. Life is complex and full of uncertainty, and any charitable giving plan you decide on will only succeed if it is part of an integrated overall estate, tax, retirement, and financial plan. Your plan should include and coordinate:

Estate Planning Documents: At minimum, you will need four key documents in your plan. These are (a) a durable power of attorney (authorizes an agent to handle tax, legal, and financial matters), (b) a health care proxy (designates an agent to make health care decisions for you), (c) a living will (a statement of your health care wishes), and (d) a will (distributes assets, appoints guardians, etc.). Depending on the nature of your plan, you may require a range of different trusts such as a revocable living trust, insurance trust, charitable remainder trust (CRT), charitable lead trust (CLT), marital trust (QTIP), and so on.

Investment Plan: You should have an overall investment allocation plan for all your investable assets. Within that plan, each separate investment basket must be planned. Your tax-deferred accounts, such as IRAs, may have different investment allocations than a by-pass trust under your late husband's will. If you establish a charitable trust, its assets will have to be planned with appropriate consideration to the trust terms.

Life and Related Insurance: Your insurance needs, which could include life insurance, disability insurance, and long-term care insurance, should be evaluated based on your circumstances and the planning you pursue. If you donate significant assets to the Society, you might feel more inclined to opt for long-term care insurance than you may have been had you retained full control over a larger asset base. If you cannot obtain insurance because of your MS, your plan has to reflect that.

Property and Casualty Insurance: You must be certain that all property, fire, casualty, and other risks are properly addressed. This coverage is essential to protect the assets you retain. Further, insurance coverage will often have to be modified as you implement your plan. If you give commercial real estate to a charitable remainder trust CRT, that trust and its trustees should be listed as named insureds on the property and casualty insurance. Your umbrella or personal excess liability coverage must be coordinated with the ownership and size of your assets.

Tax Returns and Planning: Your accountant should be certain that all applicable tax returns (income, gift, estate, etc.) are filed. Ongoing tax planning will often be required to address changes in facts or the law.

Implement Your Plan

So, now you've identified the people, assets, and goals important to you. You have developed a comprehensive plan with an integrated planning team—it's time to pull the trigger and implement your plan. Too often, the excitement and motivation is lost when you reach the implementation stage of a plan. Don't lose sight of the end goal. It's vital that you continue your focus on the implementation of your plan. You need to follow up with all your advisers to be certain that they are all in agreement with the plan and understand their respective roles. Regardless of the roles you believe any of your advisers are taking, you should be certain that all aspects of your plan are implemented, all documents signed, all accounts opened, and all other issues dealt with.

Monitor Your Plan

Most charitable planning techniques will require periodic monitoring to ensure that they are being handled properly. The following is a partial checklist for many of the techniques noted in this book. However, you should assemble your own personalized checklist with your advisers for your exact plan.

Bequest Under Your Will

If you make a bequest in your will to the Society, that bequest should periodically be monitored. The following are some of the possible steps you should review with your advisers:

- The Society should be properly named: National Multiple Sclerosis Society, doing business at 733 Third Avenue, New York, New York 10017.
- The Society should be notified of the bequest.
- The Society should review the language to be certain it will achieve your intended goal.
- You should sign a pledge card backing up the bequest.
- Your overall financial and estate plan should be reviewed annually to be certain that the size of the bequest to the Society is consistent with your current goals, net worth, and other factors.

- If your bequest was specific as to the application of the dollars to be given, such as for a specific research goal, you must confirm that the narrowness is still appropriate in light of new developments. MS research is dynamic. It would be unfortunate to create legal entanglements by leaving a bequest for a specific type of research that is no longer relevant.

Charitable Lead Trust

A CLT provides a distribution during its term to the Society, and thereafter funds are distributed to your designated heirs. The following are some of the monitoring steps that you should review with your advisers:

- The trust document creating the CLT must be properly signed.
- Your advisers must determine whether the trust is to be taxed as a grantor trust or non-grantor trust.
- A tax identification number (TIN) must be obtained from the IRS.
- Assets you've identified for contribution to the CLT must be transferred.
- CLT assets must be invested in a manner that comports with the goals of your plan.
- Your accountant must file an annual tax return (the type of which will depend on the manner in which your CLT was planned).

- If your CLT is a charitable lead uni-trust (CLUT) the trust assets must be valued each year.
- Periodic distributions to the Society (at least annually, but perhaps more frequently) must be made as required in the CLT.
- Depending on your agreement with the Society, there may be involvement with major gift professionals each year as to the use of the funds being donated.
- Investment performance must be monitored.
- Annual records of all trust activities must be kept by the trustee.
- Depending on the terms of the trust document and state law, the trustees may have certain reporting obligations to the beneficiaries.
- When the trust term ends, the assets must be distributed to your heirs (or in many cases to further trusts to protect them), the trust agreement must terminate, a final tax return must be filed, and other housekeeping actions taken.

Charitable Remainder Trust

A CRT provides a distribution during its term to you and possibly to other named beneficiaries. After the trust term, the Society receives the trust assets. You will obtain an income tax deduction on the donation to the CRT. The following are some of the monitoring steps that you should review with your advisers:

- The trust document creating the CRT must be properly signed. Your advisers must verify that the 50%, 10%, and other tests discussed in Chapter 6 are met.
- A tax identification number (TIN) must be obtained from the IRS.
- Assets you've identified for contribution to the CRT must be transferred.
- Any unique nuances of those assets must be considered and planned for. For example, if you transfer real estate to a CRT the trustees and/or the Society may require a title report, environmental inspection, and other steps to protect the CRT. Property and casualty insurance must be amended to list the trust and trustees as named insureds.
- If you've also paired your CRT with an insurance plan to replace assets for your heirs, that plan must be separately monitored.
- CRT assets must be invested in a manner that comports with the goals of your plan.
- Your accountant must file an annual tax return.
- If your CRT is a charitable remainder uni-trust (CRUT), the trust assets must be valued each year.
- Periodic distributions to the current beneficiaries (at least annually, but perhaps more frequently) must be made as required in the CRT.
- Investment performance must be monitored.
- Any unique nuances of your CRT must be monitored. If the trust is structured as a FLIP-CRUT, the event that triggers the flip in payments must be monitored. If your CRT is structured as a NIM-CRUT, as explained in Chapter 6, the make-up payments must be monitored.

- Annual records of all trust activities must be kept by the trustee.
- Depending on the terms of the trust document and state law, the trustees may have certain reporting obligations to the beneficiaries.
- When the trust term ends, the assets must be distributed to the Society, the trust agreement must terminate, a final tax return must be filed, and other housekeeping actions taken.

Donating Insurance to the Society

You can use insurance in a host of ways in your charitable plan. The simplest is to donate an insurance policy to the Society. The following are some of the monitoring steps that you should review with your advisers if you are using an insurance trust in your plan:

- Have your attorney confirm that, under your state law, the Society will have the legal right to own insurance on your life (insurable interest).
- Review available insurance policy products with your insurance consultant and major gift professional from the Society.
- Apply for a permanent insurance policy to be owned by the Society.
- Contribute cash as a donation each year to the Society so that the organization can purchase the policy.
- If you are transferring an existing policy to the trust, it must be valued and all necessary assignment documents completed and filed with the insurance company issuing the policy.

- Insurance performance must be monitored. This might mean obtaining an in-force policy illustration every year and checking on the financial status of the insurance company.

Irrevocable Life Insurance Trust

Another way to use insurance in your charitable plan is to establish an irrevocable life insurance trust (ILIT) to own insurance on your life to replace assets you've given to the Society. You can simply donate a policy to the Society, or engage in other types of insurance and charitable planning discussed in this book. The checklist to monitor each of these plans will be quite different depending on the nature of your plan. The following are some of the monitoring steps that you should review with your advisers if you are using an insurance trust in your plan:

- The insurance trust document, if one is to be used, must be properly signed.
- A tax identification number (TIN) must be obtained from the IRS.
- Contribute cash at inception and usually annually thereafter to the trust to pay for insurance premiums.
- If you are transferring an existing policy to the trust, it must be valued and all necessary assignment documents completed and filed with the insurance company issuing the policy.
- Annual demand or "Crummey" power notices must be issued by your trustees to the beneficiaries in order to qualify annual gifts to the trust for the annual gift tax exclusion. Discuss this planning step with your advisers.

- Trust assets must be invested in a manner that comports with the goals of your plan. In most cases, this will be a modest amount of cash maintained in a non–interest bearing checking account.
- Insurance performance must be monitored. This might mean obtaining an in-force policy illustration periodically and checking on the financial status of the insurance company.
- Annual records of all trust activities must be kept by the trustee.
- Depending on the terms of the trust document and state law, the trustees may have certain reporting obligations to the beneficiaries.
- When the trust term ends, the assets must be distributed to the Society and any other beneficiaries, the trust agreement must terminate, a final tax return must be filed, and other housekeeping actions taken.

Monitor Your Overall Plan, Not Just One Charitable Technique

During all phases of your planning, you must be sure that each key person you've identified is protected, that assets you have are integrated into the plan in the most optimal manner, and that your plan is monitored on a regular basis to ensure that it remains on track to meet your goals. The entire process is dynamic. The people you are concerned about protecting may change over time. The circumstances affecting each of them will certainly change over time. Your assets will change. Even your goals may change as you age, mature, and new situations and circumstances evolve. A diagnosis of MS changes so many aspects of your life. Your planning must be monitored for these changes as well as the formalities listed here.

Chapter Summary

The techniques or planning ideas in this book that caught your attention were developed into components of a comprehensive plan in this chapter. Checklists and practical suggestions about how develop you own action plan help you take the next step.

This chapter explained the practical and detailed follow-up you need to really make any charitable plan work for you. Without the proper follow-up, your plan is unlikely to achieve your many personal goals.

Now that you have the ideas and action steps to take, make up your own checklist of "To Do" items, follow-up with your advisers, and begin the process of supporting the Society in its mission to find a cure, while achieving other important personal goals.

GLOSSARY

Adjusted Gross Income (AGI): Total earnings (wages, interest, dividends, rental income, etc.) of a donor reported on Form 1040 Personal Income Tax Return, reduced only by certain limited deductions (alimony, IRA contributions, etc.). AGI is the benchmark for determining when limitations are applied to deducting certain charitable contributions.

Alternative Minimum Tax (AMT): A tax calculation that limits deductions and other preferential tax benefits and may result in all your income being taxed at a flat rate that is lower than the regular tax, but with a resulting higher tax. This might result in a lower income tax benefit from a charitable gift.

Annual Exclusion: The amount that anyone can gift each year to another (other than a charity) without incurring any gift tax consequences.

Appraisal: Donations of property to charity must be supported by a formal determination of value (appraisal) that meets specified requirements of the tax laws.

Benefit: If you receive a valuable benefit that is more than a token gift (e.g., a T-shirt) in recognition of your donation, the amount of your charitable contribution deduction may have to be reduced.

Carryforward: If you cannot use a current contribution as a deduction in the current year because of limitations on your contribution deduction, you may be able to claim the unused deductions in future years.

Charitable Bail Out: In some instances, you might be able to donate stock in a closely held business or real estate venture to the Society or a charitable remainder trust (CRT), obtain a current income tax deduction, and provide a mechanism for succession planning of the business or venture.

Charitable Lead Annuity Trust: A trust that pays a fixed annuity amount in each year of its term to the Society, following which the assets of the trust are distributed to heirs of the donor, usually children.

Charitable Lead Uni-trust: A trust that pays a variable amount determined each year based on the asset value of the trust to the Society, following which the assets of the trust are distributed to the heirs of the donor, which may include children or even grandchildren.

Charitable Remainder Annuity Trust: A trust that pays a fixed percentage of the initial value of assets contributed to the trust for a specified number of years or for life. Following these interests, the Society receives the assets.

Charitable Remainder Uni-trust: A charitable trust that pays the donor a variable amount each year based on a fixed percentage (determined when the trust is established) of the value of the trust assets each year.

Child: You can benefit a child and the Society using charitable lead trusts (CLTs), making a child a current beneficiary of a charitable remainder trust (CRT) with you, and using other techniques.

Closely Held Business: A number of charitable giving techniques can benefit a closely held or family business, including donations of inventory, donations that are deductible without limitation as advertising expenses, charitable bail-outs of stock, and more.

Depreciation: The systematic deduction of the portion of the cost of building and acquiring an asset, such as a building, over a period allowed by the tax laws. If depreciable assets are donated to the Society, a portion of the deduction may be reduced based on prior depreciation deductions.

Estate Tax: A tax assessed on the value of assets and certain other rights you own at death. Outright contributions to the Society are deductible in full against the amounts subject to tax. The state where you permanently reside, as well as any state in which you own certain assets, may assess an estate tax as well as the federal government.

Fair Market Value: The value a willing buyer would pay to a willing seller with full knowledge of the transaction. While many types of donations to the Society are deductible based on the fair market value of assets you donate, other deductions are limited.

Farm: You can donate a remainder interest in a farm, you can use or live in it for your lifetime (and your spouse's if you wish) and, upon death, the property will be transferred to the Society.

Generation-skipping Transfer (GST) Tax: A tax that applies, in addition to the gift and estate tax, to multi-generational transfers made to generations below that of a donor's children, such as grandchildren.

Gift Annuity: A donor gifts property, such as appreciated stock, to the Society in exchange for specified periodic payments for life.

Gift Tax: A tax is assessed on the lifetime transfers of assets. The first $12,000 per person is excluded from gift tax (this amount is inflation adjusted), and you can gift $1 million before incurring tax. Charitable giving techniques that benefit the Society can be used to minimize gift tax impact on large transfers to your heirs.

Grandchild: Gifts or bequests to grandchildren can trigger the generation-skipping transfer (GST) tax. Incorporating charitable giving into your planning for grandchildren (and even further descendants) can enable you to minimize GST impact.

Inter-Vivos: A gift made while the donor is alive is referred to as an inter-vivos gift.

Inventory: Businesses can donate inventory items to the Society and obtain valuable tax deductions.

IRA: You can bequeath your IRA or other retirement plan accounts to the Society and save substantial income and estate taxes. A limited opportunity exists to donate up to $100,000 of your IRA to the Society while you are alive.

Itemized Deductions: You are allowed to deduct a list of possible expenditures, including charitable contributions, as deductions on your personal income tax return. The limitations on these deductions may affect the value of your charitable contribution deductions.

Life Insurance Donations: You can donate existing insurance policies or buy a new policy for the Society.

Life Insurance Replacement: You can purchase life insurance to replace the value of assets you donate to the Society so that your estate stays whole.

Mortgaged Property: If you donate mortgaged property to the Society, you will have an income tax consequence.

Partial Interest: You cannot generally obtain a deduction for donating a portion of an asset (partial interest) unless you use prescribed techniques such as a charitable remainder trust (CRT), charitable lead trust (CLT), or a remainder interest in a residence or farm.

Part Gift/Part Sale: If a donor sells an asset at a reduced favorable price to the Society, the bargain portion of the purchase price is treated as a charitable gift and the sale portion as a taxable sale.

Partial Interest: In some instances, less than all of an asset or ownership right may be contributed to the Society. There are restrictions on such contributions, so they must be planned to secure a tax deduction.

Partnership: If your partnership donates property you, as the partner, will report the charitable contribution deduction.

Part Sale/Part Gift: If real estate subject to a mortgage is donated to the Society, it is treated as if it is a part sale (based on the mortgage amount) and a donation of the balance. If a donor wants to be paid something for any property given to the Society, then part of the property will be treated as if it was sold, and part as if it was given.

Phase-Out: Itemized deductions (expenses you may deduct on your income tax return) are subject to certain phase-out rules that may limit those deductions, including charitable contributions.

Present Value: The value in current dollars of a sum to be received at some future date, or a series of payments to be received over future periods.

Private Foundation: You can form your own charity in order to maintain greater control over donations and achieve other personal and family benefits.

Property: You can donate almost any type of property to the Society. Each different asset you donate raises its own planning opportunities and issues.

QTIP: A trust that qualifies for the unlimited gift and estate tax marital deduction.

Real Estate: You can donate real estate to the Society or to a charitable remainder trust (CRT) to ultimately benefit the Society. Real estate donations, however, raise a host of issues: mortgages, environmental, title, etc.

Recapture: On the sale or donation of an asset that was depreciated, a portion or all of that depreciation may reduce the charitable contribution deduction.

Remainder Interest: The value of property at a future date, after current rights held by another. For example, a donor's spouse can be given the right to income from a trust and, on the spouse's death, a charity receives any assets left in the trust. The charity's interest is a remainder interest.

Residence: You can donate a remainder interest in your home to the Society. You can continue to reside in your home for your life (and your spouse's life, if applicable) and, on death, the Society receives your home. You can qualify for a current income tax deduction for a portion of the value of your home.

Retirement Plan: You can bequeath your retirement plan to the Society or use retirement assets to satisfy a bequest in your will and save income and estate taxes.

S Corporation: S corporation stock can be donated to the Society directly or through a charitable remainder trust (CRT). S corporations can donate inventory to the Society or deduct certain contributions as advertising expenses.

Spouse: You can combine charitable and marital planning to benefit your spouse and the Society and avoid any gift or estate taxes.

Stock: You can donate stock to the Society and receive a current income tax deduction. You can use stock to fund various types of trust to benefit the Society.

Substantiation: Donations to the Society must be documented in order to secure your tax benefits.

Testamentary: A charitable gift can be made in your will and is effective on your death; this is a testamentary gift.

Wealth Replacement Trust: You can donate assets to the Society or to a charitable remainder trust to benefit the organization and form an insurance trust (ILIT) to own insurance on your life to replace the value of the assets donated to the Society.

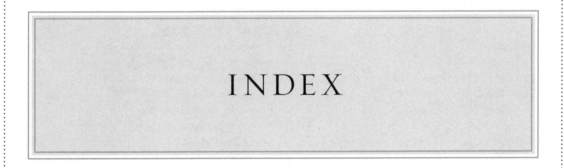

INDEX